Spectacle Lenses: Theory and Practice

Publisher: Caroline Makepeace
Development editor: Myriam Brearley
Production controller: Chris Jarvis
Desk editor: Claire Hutchins
Cover designer: Alan Studholme

Spectacle Lenses: Theory and Practice

Colin Fowler BSc PhD FCOptom

Senior Lecturer, Optometry and Vision Sciences, Aston University, Birmingham, UK

Keziah Latham Petre BSc PhD MCOptom

Lecturer, Optometry and Vision Sciences, Aston University, Birmingham, UK

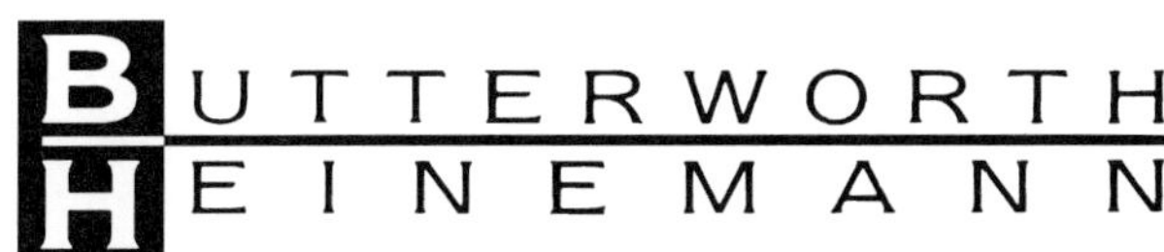

OXFORD AUCKLAND BOSTON JOHANNESBURG MELBOURNE NEW DELHI

Butterworth-Heinemann
Linacre House, Jordan Hill, Oxford OX2 8DP
225 Wildwood Avenue, Woburn, MA 01801-2041
A division of Reed Educational and Professional Publishing Ltd

 A member of the Reed Elsevier plc group

First published 2001

British Library Cataloguing in Publication Data
Fowler, Colin
Spectacle lenses: theory and practice
1. Ophthalmic lenses
I. Title I. Petre, Keziah Latham
617.7'522

Library of Congress Cataloguing in Publication Data
Fowler, Colin.
Spectacle lenses: theory and practice/Colin Fowler, Keziah Latham Petre.
p. ; cm.
Includes bibliographical references and index.
ISBN 0 7506 2370 5
1. Ophthalmic lenses. 2. Eyeglasses. I. Latham Petre, Keziah. II. Title
[DNLM: 1. Eyeglasses. 2. Optics. 3. Refractive Errors. 4. Vision. WW 354 F785s 2001]
RE976.F69 2001
617.7'522–dc21 00–054373

ISBN 0 7506 2370 5

Composition by Scribe Design, Gillingham, Kent, UK
Printed and bound in Great Britain by The Bath Press, Avon

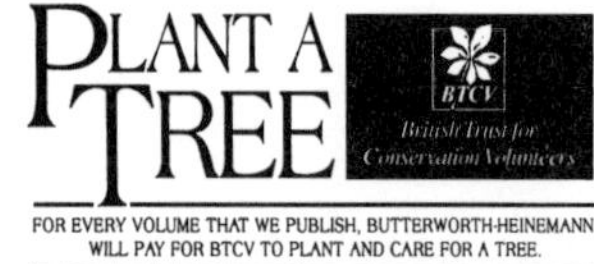

Contents

Glossary of terms

Symbol	*Meaning*	*Units*
σ	Reflectance	–
τ_v	Minimum integrated visible transmission	–
a	apical angle of a prism	degrees
a	apparent thickness	m
c	decentration from optical centre	cm
CVF	curve variation factor	–
d	deviation of a ray (= i′ – i)	degrees
DC	dioptres cylindrical power	m^{-1}
DS	dioptres spherical power	m^{-1}
f	focal length	m
F	first principal focus	–
F′	second principal focus	–
F	focal power of a thin lens	D
F_1	front surface power	D
F_2	rear surface power	D
F_e	equivalent power of thick lens/system	D
F_v	front vertex power of a thick lens	D
F'_v	back vertex power of a thick lens	D
i	angle of incidence	degrees
i'	angle of refraction	degrees
I	image	–
l	object distance (from lens to object)	m
l'	image distance (from lens to image)	m
L	incident vergence	D
L'	exit vergence	D
n	refractive index (of first material)	–
n'	refractive index (of second material)	–
O	object	–
p	conic coefficient of the surface	–
P	prism power	Δ
PF	power factor	–
r	radius of curvature	m
r_0	paraxial radius of curvature of conic surface	m
s'	sagittal image	–
SF	shape factor	–
SM	spectacle magnification	–
t	actual thickness	m
t'	tangential image	–
T	Transmission	–
z	position of centre of rotation of the eye	m

Introduction

The spectacle lens is a fascinating combination of many facets. It must be primarily utilitarian, in that it enables the wearer to see better. But at the same time the spectacle lens is now part of what is to many also a fashion statement, a pair of spectacles. Thus lenses must be cosmetically acceptable, and also durable and preferably light in weight. These requirements can often be in conflict, which is where the skill of the individual dispensing spectacles comes into play when choosing a suitable lens form.

This book arose out of lectures given to optometry undergraduate students at Aston University, but we hope that it will be of interest to all those concerned with spectacle lenses, whether as students, practitioners, in industry, or carrying out research into vision. It is written from a UK perspective, but we have tried to avoid as much as possible using trade names and descriptions which are particular to our national market.

We are very conscious of the debt of gratitude we owe to all the authors of other texts in this subject area who have shaped our knowledge and opinions. In particular the works of von Rohr, Emsley and Swaine, Bennett, and Jalie have had a special influence on us. We would also like to thank members of the ophthalmic manufacturing industry for their ever present support, in particular Essilor UK and the Norville Group. This book would not have been possible without the patience and encouragement of our publishers, where we would particularly like to thank Caroline, Zoë and Myriam.

Finally, this book is dedicated to our families without whose patience and encouragement the project would not have been possible: Carolyn, Claire, Philip and Charlie (CF), John and Ellen (KLP).

Colin Fowler and Keziah Latham Petre

Acknowledgement

Extracts from British standards in Chapters 6 and 10 are reproduced with the permission of BSI under licence number 2000SK/0559. Complete standards can be obtained from BSI Customer Services, 389 Chiswick High Road, London W4 4AL.

1

Basic optical principles

Introduction

The purpose of a spectacle lens is to alter the path of light passing through it, generally in order to correct some error of the eyes. For theoretical calculations on ophthalmic lenses, we mostly assume that light acts in the form of *rays* and travels in straight lines. Optical diagrams assume that incident light travels from left to right. The path of a ray of light is described by its *vergence*. Vergence is defined as the reciprocal of the distance in metres from a plane of interest (e.g. A in Figure 1.1) to the focal point (F in Figure 1.1). The unit of vergence is therefore m^{-1}. Although not an SI unit, values in reciprocal metres are generally called *dioptres*, abbreviated to D. In Figure 1.1a, the parallel rays of light in the first diagram have zero vergence, as the separation between the rays remains constant throughout the rays' path. In this case, the distance to the focal point is infinite and the reciprocal value, giving the vergence, is zero. In Figure 1.1b, the rays of light are converging towards a focus and have a positive vergence. The vergence of the light at point A is 1/+1, or +1 D. At B, the distance from the point of interest to the focal point has reduced to 0.5 m, so the vergence increases to 1/+0.5, or +2 D. At C, 0.25 m from the focal point, the vergence is +4 D. In Figure 1.1c, the separation between the rays is increasing. The rays of light are diverging from the focal point, and so the light has a negative vergence.

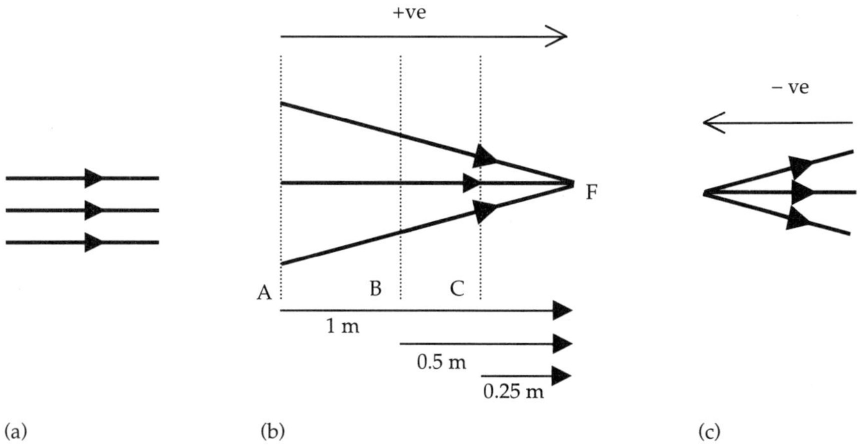

Figure 1.1. Rays of light (a) in parallel; (b) diverging; (c) converging.

For calculation purposes, we use the Cartesian sign convention. When measured relative to a refracting or reflecting surface:

- distances to the left are negative
- distances to the right are positive
- distances above the optical axis are positive
- distances below the optical axis are negative.

If an object is at a distance l from a lens, we would normally describe this in terms of the *incident vergence*, which is $1/l$. If the distance l is in metres, then the reciprocal value is indicated by the equivalent capital letter, here L, with units D.

Example

In Figure 1.2, an *object* (O) is placed 0.5 m in front of a lens. The distance would be inserted as –0.5 into a calculation, since the sign convention measures the distance *from* the optical system *to* the object, and a leftwards direction is negative. The *object distance* is given the symbol l. The incident vergence L is then $1/(-0.5) = -2$ D. After refraction by the lens, an *image* (I) is formed 1 m to the right of the lens. For calculation, this value would be given as +1. The *image distance* is given the symbol l'. The *exit vergence* from the lens is then described as $1/l'$ or L'. As a general rule, all terms associated with an object are given letter symbols on their own, e.g. l, L, whilst the equivalent terms associated with an image have a dash following them, e.g. l', L'.

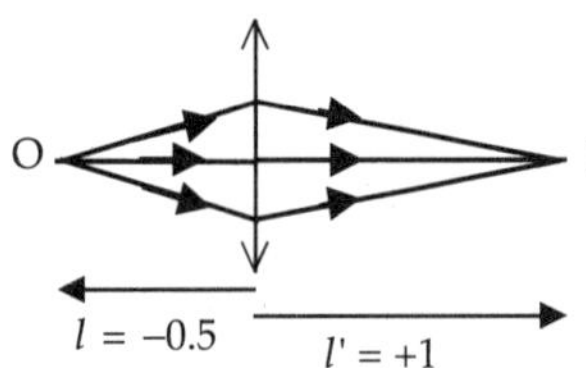

Figure 1.2. Rays of light from an object (O) are refracted by a lens and brought to focus as an image (I).

There is also a sign convention for angles, as shown in Figure 1.3. Angles measured anticlockwise are positive, and those measured clockwise are negative. The direction is taken from the normal to a ray, or from ray to axis. A *normal* is a line perpendicular to the surface at the point of reflection or refraction. The *optical axis* is a line perpendicular to the surface that passes through the physical centre of the lens, termed the *optical centre*. A further assumption about geometric optics is that light is reversible along its own path.

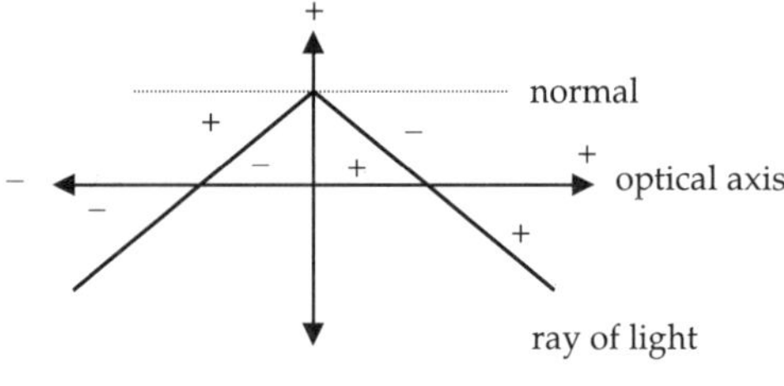

Figure 1.3. Sign convention for optical constructions.

Laws of refraction and reflection

Figure 1.4 shows a ray of light incident on a surface. The angle of incidence (i), the angle of refraction (i'), and the angle of reflection (i'') are shown.

When a ray of light meets a change of refractive index, its vergence is changed in that it will be either *refracted* (bent) or *reflected* (sent back in the same direction, usually along a different path). The angle between the incident ray and the normal is known as *the angle of incidence* (i in Figure 1.4), and the angle between the reflected or refracted ray and the normal is known either as the angle of reflection or the *angle of refraction* (i'' and i' respectively in Figure 1.4) as appropriate. Note that:

1. Incident ray, normal, and refracted/reflected ray all lie in the same plane.
2. In a mirror or reflecting surface, the angle of incidence = angle of reflection. In the diagram, $i = i'$.

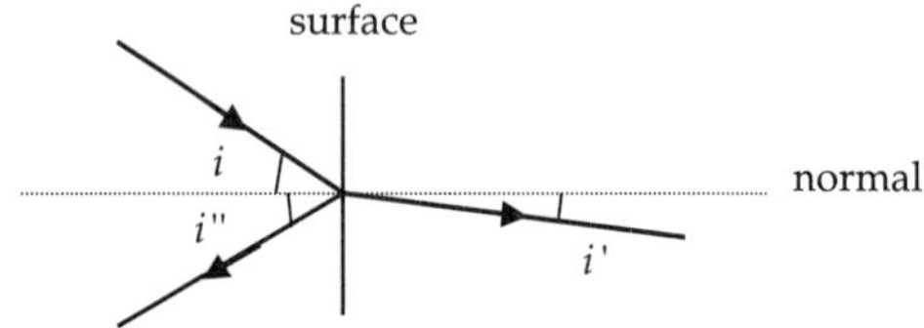

Figure 1.4. Angles of refraction and reflection at a plane (flat) surface.

3. For a refracting surface, the relation between the angle of incidence and refraction is given by *Snell's law* (see below).
4. In a plane mirror, the image is formed at the same distance behind the mirror as the object is in front.

Refractive index

The *refractive index* of a lens material is an indication of how much it bends light in the yellow–green region of the spectrum (sometimes called the mean refractive index), and is defined as the velocity of light *in vacuo* divided by the velocity of light in the material. In practice, the refractive index is measured in air, and for spectacle lenses the difference in refractive index between that measured in air and that measured *in vacuo* is insignificant. The refractive index of a medium is given the symbol n.

Refraction at a plane surface

In Figure 1.5, a beam of light meets a plane (or flat) refracting surface which separates a rarer medium of refractive index n from a denser medium of refractive index n'. Note that the emergent ray is refracted towards the normal. The same effect is seen if a stick is held in a pond at an angle; the stick appears to bend towards vertical at the pond surface. From the definition of refractive index given previously,

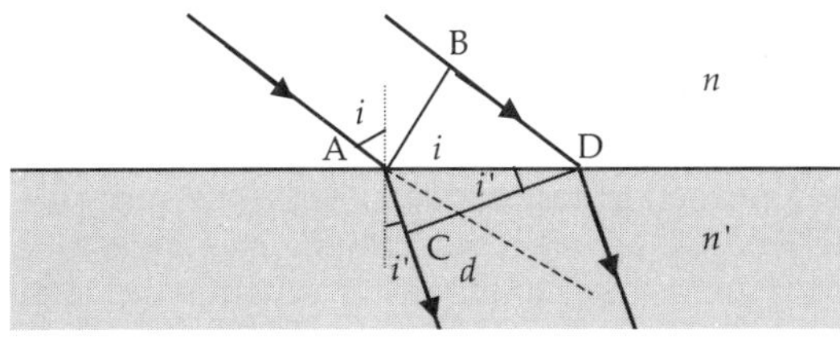

Figure 1.5. Refraction at a plane surface.

velocity of light in air = $n \times$ velocity of light in material

So, BD n = AC n'

If i is the angle of incidence at the surface and i' the angle of refraction, both angles measured relative to a normal to the surface, then from the geometry of the figure,

$\angle BAD = i$ and $\angle ADC = i'$

From trigonometry

$BD = AD \sin i$ and $AC = AD \sin i'$

then by substitution

$AD\, n \sin i = AD\, n' \sin i'$

This expression reduces to:

$n \sin i = n' \sin i'$ *Equation 1.01*

This very important relationship is known as *Snell's law.*

Note that in Figure 1.5, the angle d represents the *deviation* of the ray on refraction.

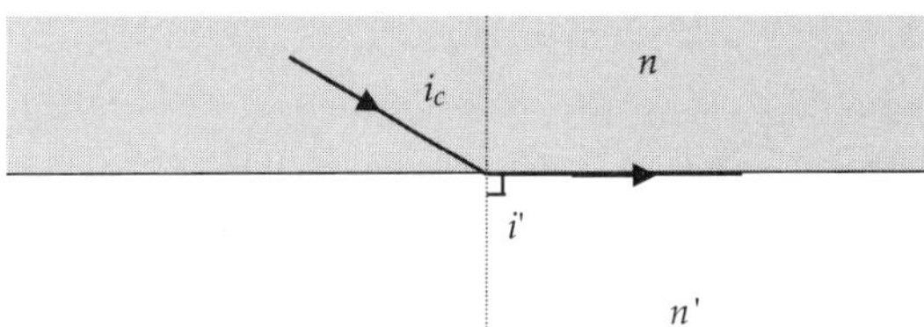

Figure 1.6. The critical angle of refraction.

Snell's law does not describe refraction for all angles. If we use the fact that light is reversible along its own path, and consider a ray of light moving from the denser material to the rarer material, as in Figure 1.6, then there will be an angle (i_c) at which light emerges parallel to the surface, with a value of i' of 90°, and $\sin i' = 1.0$. The incident angle at which this occurs is given by:

$n \sin i_c = n' 1.0$

thus

$$\sin i_c = \frac{n'}{n}$$

This special case of angle i_c is known as the *critical angle.* For the case of glass having a refractive index of 1.5 (n) in air of index 1.0 (n'), the sine of the critical angle has a value of 1/1.5, or 0.667. This is equivalent to a critical angle of 41.8°. Light striking a surface with an angle of incidence greater than the critical angle will be totally internally reflected.

Real and apparent thickness

Light travels more slowly through lens materials than through air, by the definition of refractive index. In Figure 1.7, a block of transparent material of refractive index n' has a ray of light incident to it from a rarer medium of index n. The angle of incidence is

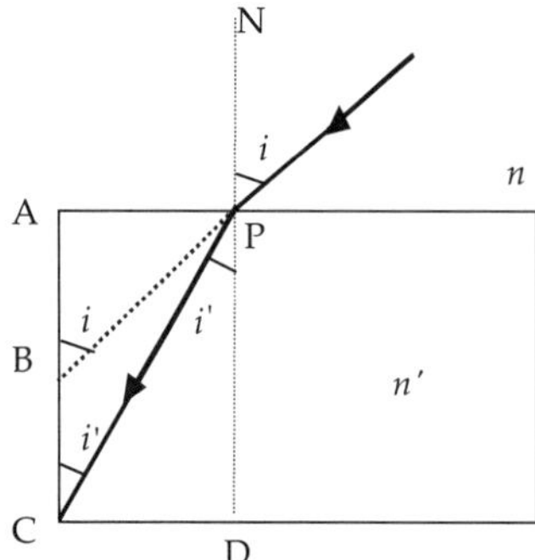

Figure 1.7. Real (AC) and apparent (AB) thickness of a plane block.

i, and if the incident ray is continued to point B, then the *apparent thickness* of the block is AB, as opposed to the *true thickness* AC. Returning to the pond analogy, a body of water will appear to be shallower than it actually is when viewed from above. From the geometry of Figure 1.7,

$$\tan i = \frac{AP}{AB} \text{ and } \tan i' = \frac{AP}{AC}$$

If we consider the angles to be small (in practice, about 5°), then the sine of any angle, the tangent, and the value of the angle itself in radians are all very similar. Thus from Snell's law,

$$n\, i = n'\, i'$$

and if the true thickness AC is given by t, and the apparent thickness AB by a, then

$$\frac{AP}{a} n = \frac{AP}{t} n'$$

$$\frac{n}{a} = \frac{n'}{t}$$

$$a = \frac{t}{n'} n$$

Since n is usually air and hence has a practical value of unity, this reduces to:

$$a = \frac{t}{n'} \qquad \textit{Equation 1.02}$$

Refraction at a curved surface

Whilst knowledge of refraction at a plane surface is important, most spectacle lenses will have curved surfaces. Figure 1.8 shows a convex spherical refracting surface, with a *radius of curvature* of r, which has a centre of curvature at C. A point on the axis (A) is imaged on the axis (A′). Incident light is in a rarer medium of refractive index n, and the denser medium has a refractive index of n'. The object and image distances from the surface are l and l' respectively. The ray intersects the surface at a point P, which is y metres above the axis of symmetry.

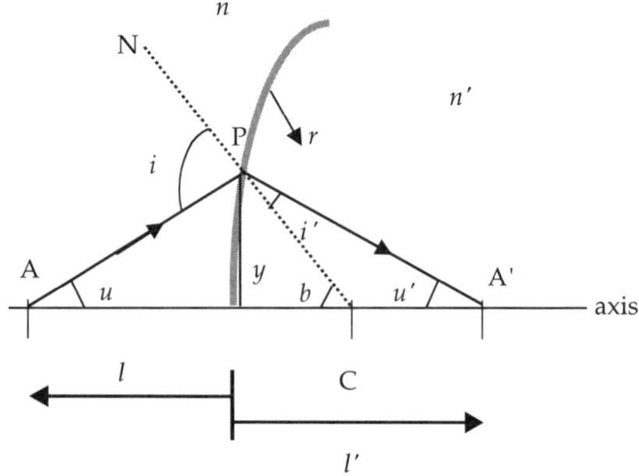

Figure 1.8. Refraction at a curved surface.

As mentioned earlier, the angles of incidence and refraction are coded positive or negative, depending on whether the angle is measured from the normal to the ray in an anti-clockwise (+) or a clockwise direction (–). In the above diagram, both angles i and i' are thus positive, u' is positive and u is negative. Although the diagram has been exaggerated, the ray in practice would be *paraxial*, in that all rays are close to the axis and all the angles would be considered to be small. Hence the relationship

angle (x) in radians = $\sin x = \tan x$

can be used.

Consider ΔAPC:

$-u + b + (180 - i) = 180$

(Remember the sign convention) so

$i = b - u$

and in ΔPCA′:

$u' + i' + (180 - b) = 180$

so

$i' = b - u'$

For small angles, Snell's law can be written as

$ni = n'i'$

Since angle = tangent of angle, combining the three equations derived above gives:

$$n\left(\frac{y}{r} - \frac{y}{l}\right) = n'\left(\frac{y}{r} - \frac{y}{l'}\right)$$

$$\frac{(n' - n)}{r} = \frac{n'}{l'} - \frac{n}{l}$$

This is a useful relationship. The value $(n' - n)/r$ is described as the *power* of a surface, or more specifically as *surface power*, and is designated by F.

$$F = \frac{(n' - n)}{r} \quad \textit{Equation 1.03}$$

Similarly, n/l is known as the incident vergence (L)

$$L = \frac{n}{l} \quad \textit{Equation 1.04}$$

and n'/l' as the emergent (or exit) vergence (L')

$$L' = \frac{n'}{l'} \quad \textit{Equation 1.05}$$

all distances in metres. Thus the relationship simplifies to:

$$F = L' - L \quad \textit{Equation 1.06}$$

In other words, the power of the surface is equal to the difference between the exit and incident vergences. Put another way, the exit vergence from a surface is equivalent to the incident vergence modified by the addition of the power of the surface, or

$L' = L + F$

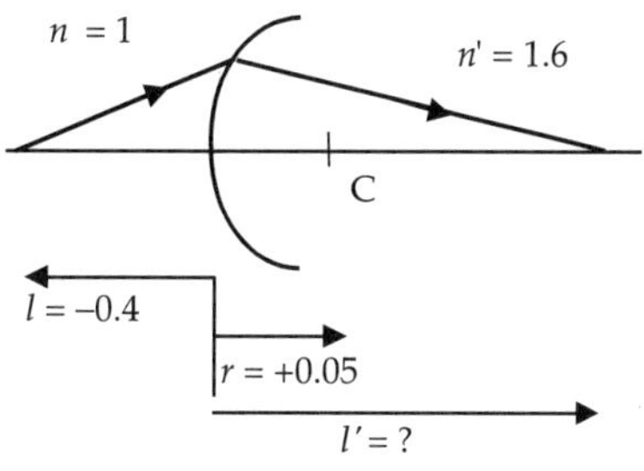

Figure 1.9. Refraction at a curved surface, numerical example.

Example

A refracting surface (in air) of refractive index 1.6 and radius of +50 mm is used to image a point in air –400 mm from the surface. Where is the image produced?

Values should be given in metres. Therefore, as shown in Figure 1.9, $l = -0.4$, $r = +0.05$, $n' = 1.6$ and $n = 1$.

From

$$\frac{(n' - n)}{r} = \frac{n'}{l'} - \frac{n}{l}$$

$$\frac{(1.6 - 1.0)}{+0.05} = \frac{1.6}{l'} - \frac{1.0}{-0.4}$$

So

$$+120 = \frac{1.6}{l'} + 2.5$$

Therefore, the surface power (F) is +12.00 D, and the incident vergence (L) is +2.50 D.

$l' = +0.168$ m

The plus sign indicates that the image is formed to the right of the refracting surface, at a distance of 168 mm.

If the incident light is parallel to the axis, as in Figure 1.10, then this indicates that the

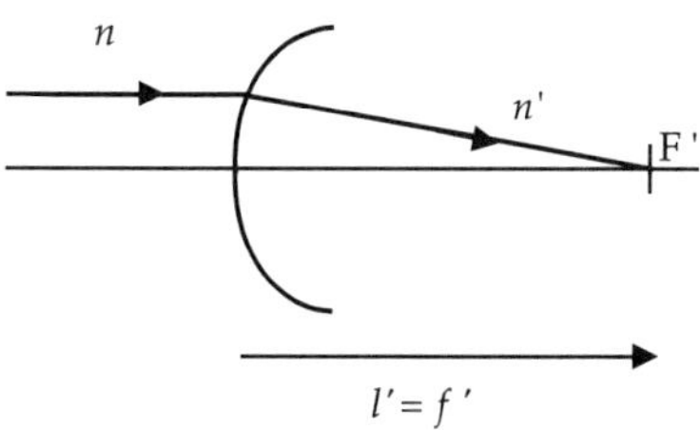

Figure 1.10. Refraction of parallel incident light by a positive curved surface.

object is at infinity. In this case, $n/l = 0$, and l' is replaced by f'. Hence the relationship

$$\frac{(n'-n)}{r} = \frac{n'}{l'} - \frac{n}{l}$$

reduces to

$$\frac{n'-n}{r} = \frac{n'}{f'} = F'$$

in this special case. F' is the power of the surface, and f' is the second principal *focal length*. The position given by F′ is the *second principal focus*.

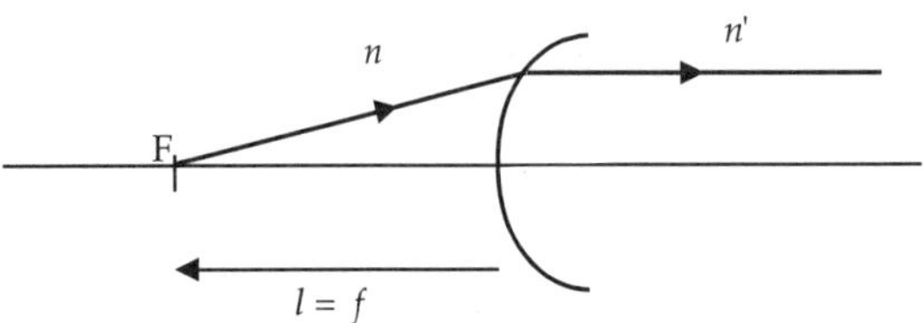

Figure 1.11. Refraction of incident light imaged at infinity by a positive curved surface.

Similarly, if the image is at infinity,

$$\frac{n'-n}{r} = -\frac{n}{f} = F$$

In this case, F is the power of the surface and f is the first principal focal length. The position of F is the *first principal focus* (Figure 1.11).

Figures 1.10 and 1.11 show convex (or converging, or positive) surfaces. Equivalent diagrams for concave (or diverging, or negative) surfaces are shown in Figure 1.12. Notice that for the concave surface the second principal focus, F′, is in front of the surface and the first principal focus, F, is behind the surface.

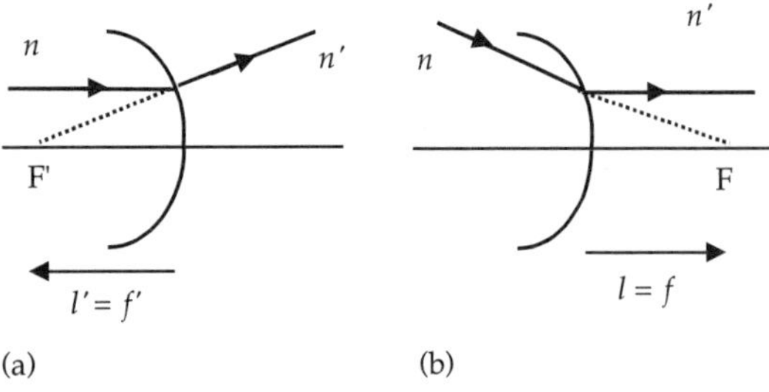

Figure 1.12. Refraction at a negative curved surface for light (a) from an object at infinity, and (b) imaged at infinity.

Lenses

So far, we have only considered refraction at one surface. Usually in spectacle lenses, we are interested in what happens when light is imaged by a lens with two surfaces.

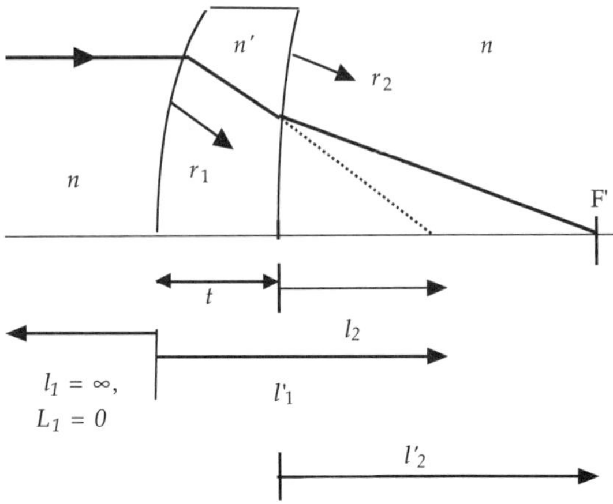

Figure 1.13. Refraction by a lens.

Let us consider first of all the special case where light is incident from a distant object, and so is parallel to the axis. As we are considering refraction at two surfaces, suffixes are used to indicate the first and second surfaces.

At the first surface:

$$L'_1 - L_1 = F_1$$

as $L_1 = 0$,

$$L'_1 = F_1$$

At the second surface:

$$L_2 = \frac{n'}{l_2}$$

The object distance for the second surface, l_2, is the distance from the lens surface to the point at which the light would come to a focus, if it were not altered by the second surface. Therefore,

$$L_2 = \frac{n'}{l'_1 - t} = \frac{n'}{(n'/F_1 - t)}$$

Dividing everything through by n'/F_1 gives:

$$L_2 = \frac{F_1}{\left\{1 - \left[\left(\frac{t}{n'}\right)F_1\right]\right\}}$$

At the second surface, the change in vergence is given by:

$L'_2 - L_2 = F_2$

Substituting the expression for L_2 into the equation above gives an expression for L'_2, the exit vergence from the rear surface of the lens. In this special case for incident light from a distant object, L'_2 is known as the *back vertex power* (BVP), and is designated as F'_v

$$F'_v = \frac{F_1}{\left\{1 - \left[\left(\frac{t}{n'}\right)F_1\right]\right\}} + F_2 \qquad \textit{Equation 1.07}$$

The back vertex power is essentially the dioptric distance from the rear surface of the lens to the second principal focal point, F′. In the case of a spectacle lens, it represents the power of the lens from the perspective of the person wearing the lens, i.e. viewing from the rear side of the lens.

Similarly, light from an object placed at the first principal focus, F, of a lens will emerge in parallel from the rear surface of the lens. In this special case the *front vertex power* (FVP) is calculated from:

$$F_v = \frac{F_2}{\left\{1 - \left[\left(\frac{t}{n'}\right)F_2\right]\right\}} + F_1 \qquad \textit{Equation 1.08}$$

The front vertex power, F_v, of the lens is of less immediate importance to the spectacle lens wearer, since it represents the power of the lens when viewed from the front surface. Looking at the equations for F_v and F'_v, however, it should be apparent that the two values will be similar unless t, the thickness of the lens, is substantial.

Example

A lens has a front surface radius of +200 mm, a rear surface radius of +200 mm, and an axial centre thickness of 5 mm. The refractive index of the lens material is 1.5.

Front surface power

$$F_1 = \frac{n' - n}{r_1} = \frac{1.5 - 1.0}{0.2} = +2.5$$

Rear surface power

$$F_2 = \frac{n - n'}{r_2} = \frac{1.0 - 1.5}{0.2} = -2.5$$

Back vertex power = +0.021 D

Note that if $F_1 = 0$, then the BVP = F_2, irrespective of thickness, since the light is not refracted at the first surface of the lens.

By no means all objects viewed through a lens will be at infinity. The positions of object and image in relation to a thick lens can be calculated in a number of different ways. The tabulated example gives two different techniques for calculating the distance of an image from the rear surface of a thick lens, for a finite object distance.

Thick lens calculation:

		Example A	*Example B*
Step along method			
Surrounding index	n	1.00	1.00
Lens index	n'	1.50	1.70
Lens thickness	t	6.00	1.00
Object distance	l_1	−200.00	−300.00
Front surface radius (mm)	r_1	50.00	200.00
Rear surface radius (mm)	r_2	200.00	50.00
At first surface:			
Incident vergence $L_1 = 1000n/l_1$		−5.00	−3.33
Front surface power (D) $F_1 = 1000(n' - n)/r_1$		10.00	3.50
Image vergence (D) $L'_1 = L_1 + F_1$		5.00	0.17
Image distance (mm) $l'_1 = 1000n'/L'_1$		300.00	10 200.00
Next object distance $l_2 = l'_1 - t$		294.00	10 199.00
At second surface:			
Incident vergence (D) $L_2 = 1000n'/l_2$		5.10	0.17
Rear surface power (D) $F_2 = 1000(n-n')/r_2$		−2.50	−14.00
Image vergence $L'_2 = L_2 + F_2$		**2.60**	**−13.83**
Image distance (mm) $l'_2 = 1000n/L'_2$		384.31	−72.29
Formula method			
Use back vertex power formula, but rather than F_1, use $(L_1 + F_1)$. Thus, assuming lens in air			
$L_1 + F_1$		5.00	0.17
Image vergence (D) $L'_2 = F_1/(1-(t/n')F_1) + F_2$ *(note that* t *is in metres)*		**2.60**	**−13.83**

One method uses the so called 'step along' technique, where the change of vergence is calculated for light at each surface as it passes through the lens, and the second uses an adaptation of the back vertex power formula.

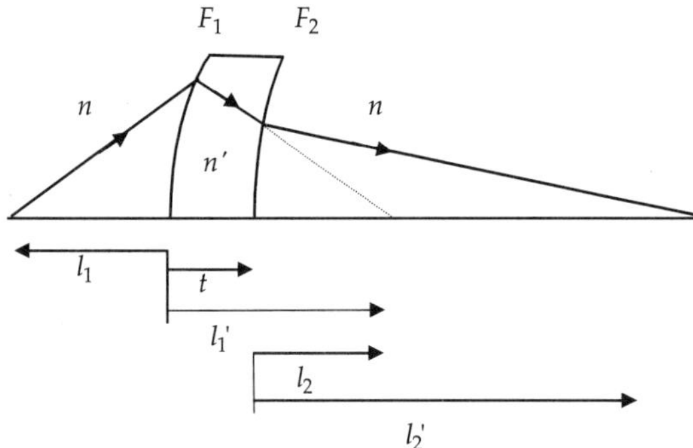

Figure 1.14. Refraction by a lens of an object not at infinity.

Consider Example A. A lens of refractive index 1.5 and thickness 6 mm is used in air. The radius of curvature of the front surface is +50 mm and the rear surface radius of curvature is +200 mm. If an object is placed 200 mm in front of the lens, where is the image located?

By the step-along method, the vergence is calculated at each surface. The image is formed 384.31 mm to the right of the second surface.

Note that distance values should be substituted into equations in metres. If millimetres are quoted, then they must be converted to metres by dividing by 1000, as shown below in two different ways for the power of the first surface, F_1.

$$F_1 = \frac{n' - n}{r} = \frac{(1.5 - 1)}{50 \times 10^{-3}} = +10$$

or,

$$F_1 = \frac{1000 \times (1.5 - 1)}{50} = +10$$

The alternative method for solving the problem is to use the back vertex power formula. The formula has to be adapted, since it is assumed in the formula that the incident vergence on the first surface is zero, i.e. light is from a distant object. Therefore the parameter F_1 in the original formula, the first surface power, is instead considered as $(L_1 + F_1)$, the vergence of light after refraction by the first surface, thereby accounting for the position of the object.

Note that such calculations can be very readily carried out using a computer spreadsheet, and indeed the accompanying table was produced in this way. This enables the effects of changes in the input variables to be quickly seen.

Thin lenses

So far, lenses have been considered with finite thickness. If we were able to neglect thickness, the expressions for BVP, FVP and equivalent power would all reduce to:

$$F = F_1 + F_2 \qquad \textit{Equation 1.09}$$

In other words, the power of a thin lens is equivalent to the sum of the front and rear surface powers. We can also produce an expression that will give object and image distances relative to a thin lens. If we take the expression for a lens *surface* and apply this to both surfaces of a lens, then at the front surface:

$$F = L' - L$$

$$\frac{n' - n}{r_1} = \frac{n'}{l'_1} - \frac{n}{l_1}$$

and at the rear:

$$\frac{n - n'}{r_2} = \frac{n}{l'_2} - \frac{n'}{l_2}$$

If the lens is thin, then t is negligible, and

$$\frac{n'}{l'_1} = \frac{n'}{l_2}$$

so

$$\frac{n' - n}{r_1} + \frac{n}{l_1} = \frac{n}{l'_2} - \frac{n - n'}{r_2}$$

$$\frac{n}{l'_2} - \frac{n}{l_1} = \frac{n' - n}{r_1} + \frac{n - n'}{r_2} = F_1 + F_2$$

this further simplifies to:

$$\frac{n}{l'} - \frac{n}{l} = F = \frac{n}{f}$$

Normally the lens is in air, so that n has a practical value of unity. Thus:

$$\frac{1}{l'} - \frac{1}{l} = \frac{1}{f}$$

This relationship enables the object and image distances from a thin lens to be calculated.

As an example, if we were to take the values in A above, but treat the lens as thin, then:

$$\frac{n'-n}{r_1} + \frac{n-n'}{r_2} = F$$

For the values in Example A this reduces to:

$$+10.00 + (-2.50) = +7.50$$

$$\frac{1}{l'} - \frac{1}{l} = \frac{1}{f}$$

$$\frac{1}{l'} - \frac{1}{-0.2} = 7.5$$

$$\frac{1}{l'} - (-5.00) = 7.50$$

$$l' = \frac{1}{2.50} = 0.4 \text{ m} = 400 \text{ mm}$$

This should be compared with the 384.31 mm from the thick lens calculation. Thus in this instance the thin lens approximation does not give a very accurate answer. However, if we reduce the lens thickness from 6.0 mm to 1.0 mm, then according to the thick lens formula the image is formed at 397.34 mm, a much closer figure to the thin lens approximation. So these approximations can be used with care, mostly with minus power lenses, which are physically thin in the centre.

Prismatic power

When Snell's law was derived earlier in this chapter, it was noted that on refraction a ray is deviated by an angle d, equal to $i' - i$. Another type of lens that can cause deviation of light is the prism. Essentially a prism is a lens consisting of two flat faces inclined to meet at some *apical angle* (a in Figure 1.15).

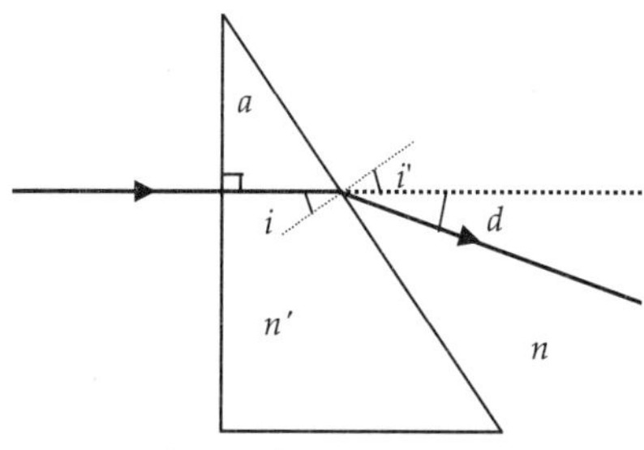

Figure 1.15. An ophthalmic, or small angle, prism.

Ophthalmic prisms are *small angle prisms*, which means that simplifications can be made in their theory. In the above diagram, a ray of light is incident normally to one face of a prism made of material of index n' with an apical angle of a. Light will pass undeviated through the first surface of the prism, but be refracted at the *second* surface according to Snell's law:

$$n' \sin i = n \sin i'$$

For small angles we can use the simplification

$$n'i = ni'$$

From the geometry of the figure, $i = a$, thus the deviation of the light, d, can be expressed as:

$$d = (i' - i)$$

$$d = (n'a - a)$$

$$d = (n' - 1)a \qquad \textit{Equation 1.10}$$

The expression derived assumes that the prism is in a surrounding medium (n) of air, and that the apical angle is less than 10°.

In ophthalmic optics, a prism is described in terms of the amount of deviation it produces, the units being *prism dioptres*. A prism with a power of 1 prism dioptre will deviate light by 1 centimetre measured at a distance of 1 metre from the prism.

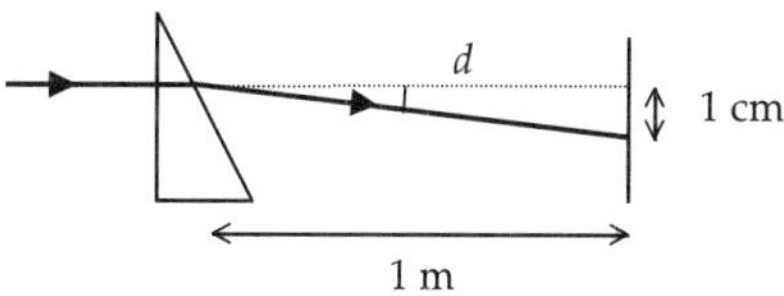

Figure 1.16. Prism of power 1 prism dioptre (1Δ).

From Figure 1.16, the tangent of the angle of deviation of a prism of power 1 prism dioptre is 1/100. Therefore, the *power of a prism*, P, in prism dioptres is 100 times the tangent of the angle of deviation. In other words,

$$P = 100 \tan d \qquad \textit{Equation 1.11}$$

The abbreviation for prism dioptre is Δ. Note that the prism dioptre is not a unit, being proportional to the tangent of the angle of deviation. It could be expressed in SI units as cm/m.

Prismatic effects of lenses

Focal lenses also have prismatic power. In a prism, all light is deviated by the same amount (Figure 1.17b), but in a lens, the deviation depends on the distance of the light ray from the optical centre of the lens (Figure 1.17a).

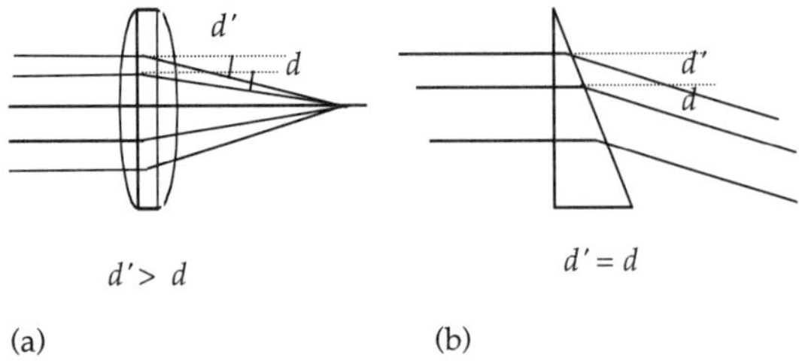

Figure 1.17. Deviation of light by (a) a lens, and (b) a prism.

The prismatic effect at any point on a lens can be defined as the power of the prism that would produce the same effect. The lens can be thought of as a series of prisms whose powers increase from zero at the optical centre to a maximum at the periphery of the lens.

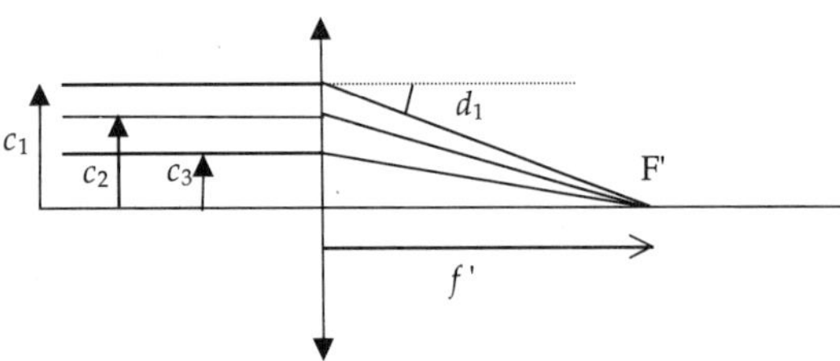

Figure 1.18. Deviation of light by a lens.

To prove how much deviation or prismatic power a lens produces, consider the following. In Figure 1.18, light from a distant object is entering a positive power lens from the left. Three rays are shown, at distances c_1, c_2, and c_3 from the optical centre.

From trigonometry,

$\tan d_1 = \text{O}/\text{A} = c_1/f$

$\tan d_2 = \text{O}/\text{A} = c_2/f$

Or more generally,

$\tan d = c/f$

Since we know that $\text{P} = 100 \tan d$, then

$\text{P} = 100\, c/f$

or

$\text{P} = cF$ *Equation 1.12*

where P is prism power (Δ), c is *decentration* from optical centre (in *cm*), and F is focal power (D). This is known as *Prentice's Rule.* Note that Prentice's Rule assumes that the lens has no spherical aberration. The practical upshot of Prentice's Rule is that if a patient looks through any point on a lens other than the optical centre, a prismatic effect will be induced.

Optical constructions

Now that we have defined the basic performance properties of lenses, it is frequently necessary to construct ray diagrams to visualize how a lens images an object. Geometric optical diagrams are useful for predicting the performance of a lens or mirror. Drawings can be to scale or schematic. Rules for diagrams are as follows, and are shown in Figure 1.19.

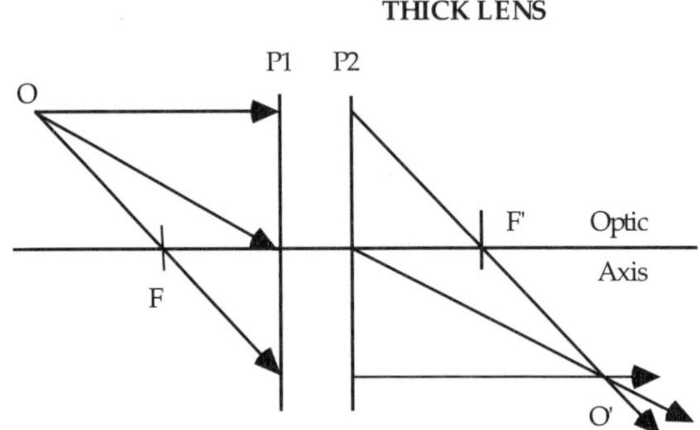

Figure 1.19. Rules of optical construction for thick lenses.

1. A ray from an object parallel to the optic axis will emerge from the system and pass through the second principal focus.
2. A ray from an object passing through the first principal focus will emerge from the system parallel to the axis.
3. A ray crossing the axis at the first principal plane will emerge parallel from the second principal plane.

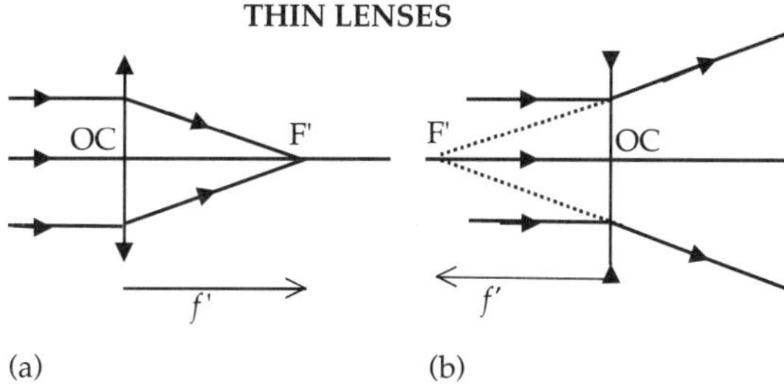

Figure 1.20. Rules of optical construction for thin lenses.

In thin lenses the principal planes coincide, and the point at which the single principal plane crosses the optic axis is known as the *optical centre* of the lens.

A thin lens is drawn as a single line with triangles at each end showing whether the lens is positive or negative by indicating the thickest part of the lens. Positive (or convex) lenses converge rays of light to the second principal focus (Figure 1.20a); negative (or concave) lenses diverge rays of light (Figure 1.20b).

For the positive lens the rays of light meet at F′, producing a *real* image. In contrast, for the negative lens the rays of light never actually meet but appear to have originated from F′. The negative lens is therefore said to produce a *virtual* image, or one that cannot be formed on a screen.

Equivalent lens power

The equivalent power of a thick lens or lens system is the power of the thin lens that could be used as an optical replacement. In Figure 1.21 two thin lenses, F_1 and F_2, are separated by a distance d. A ray of light, parallel to the axis, is incident to the system at a distance of y_1 from the axis. The second principal focus is at F′, and the angle of deviation between the incident and emergent light is p_e. If the distances are in metres, then the angles of deviation can be expressed in prism dioptres by use of Prentice's Rule (Equation 1.12) as:

$$p_1 = y_1F_1$$

$$p_2 = y_2F_2$$

but also

$$p_1 = \frac{y_1 - y_2}{d}$$

thus

$$y_1F_1 = \frac{y_1 - y_2}{d}$$

and $y_2 = y_1 - dy_1F_1$.

Since $p_e = p_1 + p_2$,

$$p_e = y_1F_1 + (y_1 - dy_1F_1)F_2$$

Also,

$$p_e = y_1F_e$$

thus,

$$y_1F_e = y_1F_1 + y_1F_2 - dy_1F_1F_2$$

Thus

$$F_e = F_1 + F_2 - dF_1F_2 \qquad \textit{Equation 1.13}$$

The *equivalent power* of the lens system, or the power of the equivalent thin lens needed to replace the lens system, is given by F_e in Equation 1.12 above. The equivalent thin lens is placed in the second principal plane of the

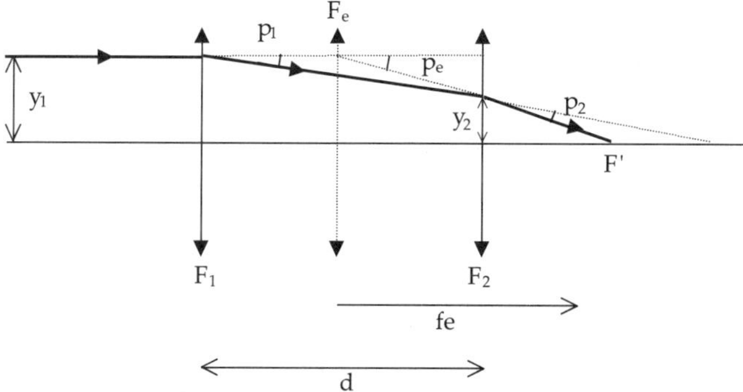

Figure 1.21. A system of thin lenses showing the position of the equivalent thin lens that could replace the system.

lens system, $-1/F_e$ away from F′, the second principal focus.

For example, if two lenses of power +10 D each are separated by 20 mm, then the equivalent power F_e is +18 D. If the lens separation is large, then apparently strange results can occur. For example, if the lens separation for the same two lenses is increased to 250 mm, then the equivalent power is −5 D. The logic behind this answer can best be realized by drawing a diagram.

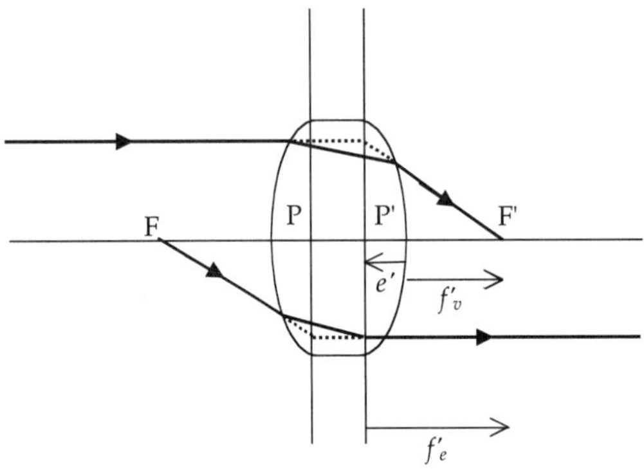

Figure 1.22. Principal planes and equivalent thin lens in a thick lens. F and F′ are the first and second focal points, respectively, and P and P′ represent the first and second principal points. The thin lens that could replace the thick lens has equivalent power F_e and is placed at P′. The distance from the rear lens surface to the second principal point is given by e'.

A similar form of expression can also be used to calculate the equivalent power of a thick lens in air (Figure 1.22). Substituting the expression for apparent thickness, t/n', for d in the above expression gives us

$$F_e = F_1 + F_2 - \frac{t}{n'} F_1 . F_2 \qquad \textit{Equation 1.14}$$

The position of the equivalent thin lens depends on the position of the *principal planes*. In Figure 1.22, the equivalent thin lens will be positioned in the plane of the second principal point, P′. The position of P′ relative to the rear surface of the lens (e′) is given by:

$$e' = f'_v - f'_e \qquad \textit{Equation 1.15}$$

where f'_v is the back vertex focal length and f'_e is the focal length of the equivalent thin lens. Alternatively, by combining Equation 1.14 with the back vertex power formula (Equation 1.07), the position of the second principal point is given by:

$$e' = \left(\frac{t}{n'}\right)\left(\frac{F_2}{F_e}\right) \qquad \textit{Equation 1.16}$$

Equivalent power is important in relation to the magnification properties of a lens. The position of the principal planes varies with lens form (see Chapter 3).

Curved mirrors

Although mirrors are not used in their usual sense in spectacle lenses, curved mirror theory is required when considering topics such as lens surface reflections and keratometry.

Single surface refraction formulae can be readily used for calculations on curved mirrors by simply making the refractive index after reflection minus the value for incident light. In other words in air, $n = 1$, then $n' = -1$.

$$F = \frac{n' - n}{r} = \frac{-1 - 1}{r} = \frac{-2}{r}$$

Hence, from the power of a surface:

$$f = \frac{-r}{2}$$

In other words, the focal length of a mirror is half the radius of curvature.

When constructing ray diagrams involving curved mirrors, the following rules apply:

1. A ray from object parallel to the optic axis will emerge from the system and pass through the second principal focus.
2. A ray from object passing through the first principal focus will emerge from the system parallel to the axis.
3. A ray directed towards the centre of curvature will be reflected back along its own path.
4. A ray intersecting the mirror at the vertex will be reflected at an equal angle.

Example

In Figure 1.23:

- Ray 'a' is parallel to the optic axis, and is reflected as if it came from the focal point F.

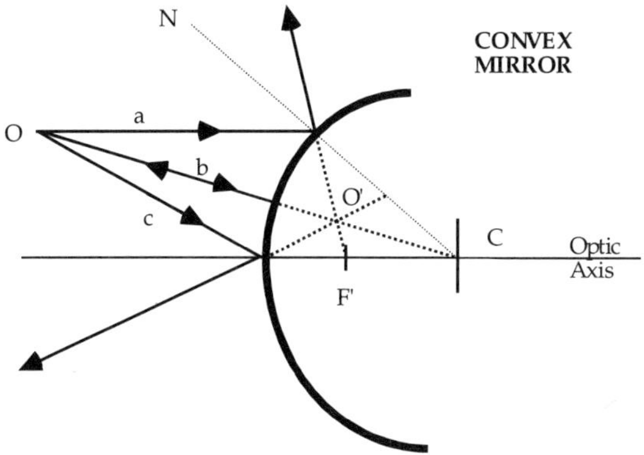

Figure 1.23. Reflection by a convex mirror.

- Ray 'b' is incident towards the centre of curvature C, and is reflected back along its own path.
- Ray 'c' intersects the mirror at the vertex (on the axis), and is reflected at an equal angle to the angle of incidence.

Reflection at convex mirror:

Object distance (mm)	l	-50.00
Mirror radius (mm)	r	8.00
Incident refractive index	n	1.00
Emergent refractive index	n'	-1.00
Power of mirror (D)	$F = 1000(n' - n)/r$	-250.00
Incident vergence (D)	$L = 1000/l$	-20.00
Exit vergence	$L' = L + F$	-270.00
Image position	$l' = 1000n'/L'$	3.70

In the above example, the image distance (l') is positive, so it is formed to the right of the mirror.

Summary

In this chapter, the basic optical principals required to understand spectacle lenses have been derived. Summarized below, listed in the order in which they occur in the text, are the formulae used in this chapter.

Formulae

Formula	*Name*	*Equation number*
$n \sin i = n' \sin i'$	Snell's law	1.01
$a = \frac{t}{n'}$	apparent thickness	1.02
$F = \frac{(n' - n)}{r}$	surface power	1.03
$L = \frac{n}{l}$	incident vergence	1.04
$L' = \frac{n'}{l'}$	exit vergence	1.05
$F = L' - L$	power of a surface	1.06
$F'_v = \frac{F_1}{\left\{1 - \left[\left(\frac{t}{n'}\right)F_1\right]\right\}} + F_2$	back vertex power formula	1.07
$F_v = \frac{F_2}{\left\{1 - \left[\left(\frac{t}{n'}\right)F_2\right]\right\}} + F_1$	front vertex power formula	1.08
$F = F_1 + F_2$ where		
$F + \frac{1}{f'}, F_1 = \frac{1}{l}, F_2 = \frac{1}{l'}$	thin lens formula	1.09
$d = (n' - 1)a$	deviation of light by a prism	1.10
$P = 100 \tan d$	prism power	1.11
$P = cF$	Prentice's Rule	1.12
$F_e = F_1 + F_2 - dF_1F_2$	equivalent power of lens system	1.13
$F_e = F_1 + F_2 - \frac{t}{n'}F_1F_2$	equivalent power of thick lens	1.14
$e' = f'_v - f'_e$	position of equivalent thin lens	1.15
$e' = \left(\frac{t}{n'}\right)\left(\frac{F_2}{F_e}\right)$	position of equivalent thin lens	1.16

Exercises

Questions

1. What is the vergence of light 50 cm away from an object?
2. The focal length of a lens is +33.33 cm. What is its power?
3. What is the focal length of a lens with a power of –4.17 D?
4. Light rays enter a lens in parallel and a virtual image is formed 40 cm in front of the lens. Calculate the lens power.
5. A lens of refractive index 1.50 has a radius of curvature of –4.00 cm. What is the power of the lens surface in air?
6. An object is positioned –70 cm from a lens of power +4 D. What is the vergence of the emergent light +30 cm from the lens?
7. An object is placed 50 cm in front of a lens with a focal length of 40 cm. Where is the image produced? Where is the image produced if the object is moved to a position 20 cm in front of the lens?
8. The surface power of a lens is +4.00 D and its radius of curvature is 22.5 cm. What is the refractive index of the lens?
9. A lens surface has a power of +10.00 D in air. What power does the lens surface have in water? (n for air = 1; n for lens = 1.523; n for water = 1.333).
10. A stick is held in a pond (n of water = 1.333) at an angle of 30° to the normal in air. What is the apparent orientation of the stick in water?
11. A frog in the same pond as in Question 10 is holding a stick so that it sticks out of the water. At what angle to the normal should the stick be held so that the image of the stick will be totally reflected at the pond surface?
12. Having finished with the stick, an observer on dry land spots the frog at the bottom of the pond. The pond is 2 m deep. How far below the surface does the frog appear to be to the observer?
13. Two thin lenses of power +10 D are placed in air, separated by 40 cm. An object is positioned –20 cm from the first lens. Where is the final image produced?
14. An image is formed 20 cm to the left of a –5 D lens. Where was the object?
15. Parallel rays of light are incident normally on the front surface of a glass lens (n = 1.523) with a front surface power of +8.00 DS. What is the vergence of the refracted rays after they have travelled through 5 mm of glass?
16. A lens has a refractive index of 1.7, a front surface radius of curvature of 50 mm and a rear surface radius of curvature of 200 mm. What are the powers of the front and rear surfaces? If the centre thickness of the lens is 3 mm, what are the front and back vertex powers of the lens?
17. Rearrange the back vertex power formula to make F_1 the subject of the equation (i.e. $F_1 = \ldots$).
18. A lens is required to measure +2.00 DS on a focimeter and is made with a back surface power of –6.00 DS and a centre thickness of 2.8 mm. Assuming n = 1.523, what front surface power is required?
19. A lens is produced which has a refractive index of 1.6, surface powers of +10.00 DS on the front and –5.00 DS on the rear, and a centre thickness of 5 mm. An object is placed 25 cm in front of the lens. Where is the image produced? What is the back vertex power of the lens? What is the front vertex power?
20. A plano-convex lens is made with a front surface power of +13.00 D and centre thickness of 10 mm. If the refractive index of the material is 1.5, what is the back vertex power of the lens?
21. A spectacle lens of 1.7 index material is required to have a prescription of +10.00 D and to have a centre thickness of 5 mm. If the lens to be used has a front surface power of +14 D, what should the back surface power be? What is the power and position of an equivalent thin lens to replace this thick lens?
22. A plano-concave lens is hand neutralized and found to have a back vertex power of –8.00 DS. The rear surface has a surface power of –5.23 DS, as measured with a lens measure calibrated for crown glass. What is the refractive index of the lens? What is the true back surface power of the lens?
23. A lens has the following parameters: back vertex power = +8.00 DS; rear surface power = –3.00 DS; centre thickness = 5 mm; refractive index = 1.5. What is the front

surface power of the lens?

24. What is the decentration required in a +6.00 DS lens to give 2Δ Base In?
25. What is the decentration required in a –6.00 DS lens to give 3Δ Base In?
26. A lens system is made up of two lenses of power +20.00 D (F_1) and +30.00 D (F_2), separated by 70 mm. Calculate the equivalent power and the back vertex power of the system.
27. An object is placed 1 m away from a convex mirror with a radius of curvature of 10 mm. Where is the image formed?

Answers

1. –2 D
2. +3.00 D
3. –0.24 m
4. –2.50 D
5. –12.50 D
6. +11.25 D
7. +2 m; –40 cm
8. 1.90
9. +3.63 D
10. 22° from the normal
11. 48.6° (or more)
12. 1.5 m
13. 20 cm to the right of the second lens
14. At infinity, to the left of the lens
15. +8.22 DS
16. F_1, +14.00 DS; F_2, –3.5 DS; F'_v, +10.85 DS; F_v, +10.52 DS.
17. $F_1 = \dfrac{F'_v - F_2}{1 - \dfrac{t}{n}(F_2 - F'_v)}$
18. +7.88 DS
19. 90 cm from rear lens surface. F'_v, +5.32 D; F_v, +5.08 D.
20. +14.22 D
21. F_2, –4.60 D; F_e, +9.59 D; e', –4.28 mm from the rear surface of the thick lens
22. $n = 1.8$; $F_2 = -8.00$ D
23. +10.61 DS
24. 0.33 cm in
25. 0.50 cm out
26. $F_e = +8.00$ DS; $F'_v = -20.00$ DS
27. 5.03 mm to the right of the mirror

2

Spherical lens forms

Introduction

This chapter will deal with the practical lens forms in which spectacle lenses are manufactured. From Chapter 1 it will be apparent that lenses with the same back vertex power can be manufactured in a wide variety of different forms. Early lenses were made in what is now known as *flat* form, whereas now the majority are produced as *curved*. The differences between these forms are defined in BS 3521 Part 1 (1991):

- *Curved lens*: a lens having one surface convex in all meridians, and one surface concave in all meridians.
- *Flat lens*: any other type of lens.

Thus it is important to remember that a flat lens does *not* have to have a plane surface. The comment concerning 'in all meridians' in the definition is to cover the case where a cylindrical correction is incorporated (see Chapter 3). Note that spherical curved form lenses are known as *meniscus* lenses. In Figure 2.1, lenses are shown in the position that they would be normally fitted, with incident light coming from the left, and the more negative curve next to the eye. Lens C is a steep meniscus form, whereas D would be classified as a shallow meniscus. Lens A is equi biconvex, both surfaces having identical curvature. Lens G is biconcave, but with a steeper rear surface compared to the front.

There are several reasons for using different forms of lens. Changing the form from flat to meniscus will usually improve the vision through the edge of the lens (Chapter 7). However, flat form lenses are generally thinner and lighter than curved forms (Chapter 5).

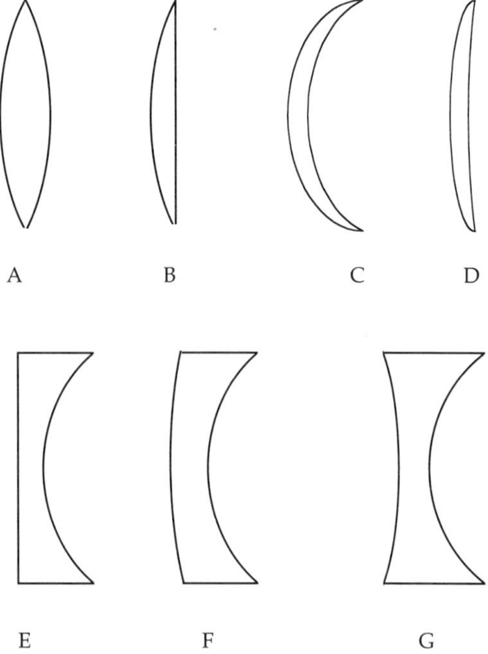

Figure 2.1. Spherical lens forms. Lenses A–D are positive, while E–G are negative. Lenses C and D are curved, having an entirely convex front surface and an entirely concave rear surface. The other lens forms are all described as flat, although only lenses B and E actually contain a plane surface.

Lens thickness

To calculate the thickness of a lens, first consider Figure 2.2. A spherical curve of radius r and centre of curvature C is cut by a chord BD. The dimension AE is known as the *sag* of the chord, and has a dimension s for a chord length of $2y$.

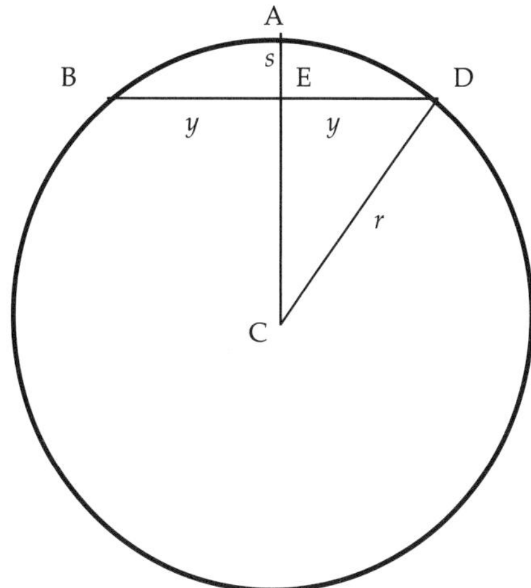

Figure 2.2. Calculation of the sag (s) of a surface. A lens surface (B–A–D) has a spherical curvature that is part of a circle of radius r and centre of curvature C. Considering a chord (B–E–D) across the lens surface, which can be considered equivalent to the lens diameter, the chord length is $2y$ and the sag of the surface (A–E) is s.

From the geometry of the figure:

$$r^2 = y^2 + (r - s)^2$$

or

$$r^2 - y^2 = (r - s)^2$$

Taking square roots of both sides of the equation, and rearranging:

$$r - s = \sqrt{(r^2 - y^2)}$$

$$s = r - \sqrt{(r^2 - y^2)} \qquad \textit{Equation 2.01}$$

In the case of r being negative, then the expression becomes:

$$s = r + \sqrt{(r^2 - y^2)}$$

From this expression, assuming that the chord length $2y$ is the same as the lens diameter, then the lens thickness can be related to the lens radius. It is also useful to have the alternative expression, solved for radius:

$$r^2 = y^2 + r^2 - 2rs + s^2$$

$$2rs = y^2 + s^2$$

$$r = (y^2 + s^2)/(2s) \qquad \textit{Equation 2.02}$$

If s is small in relation to y and r, then the value of s^2 can be ignored, so that:

$$s = y^2/(2r) \qquad \textit{Equation 2.03}$$

or

$$r = y^2/(2s) \qquad \textit{Equation 2.04}$$

Equations 2.01 and 2.02 are known as the 'exact sag' formulae, 2.03 and 2.04 being the 'approximate sag' formulae.

These sag formulae can then be used to calculate lens thickness, as shown in Table 2.1 and illustrated in Figure 2.3. The relationship of edge thickness (e) to centre thickness (t) can be derived from the expression:

$$e = t - s_1 + s_2 \qquad \textit{Equation 2.05}$$

where s_1 is the sag of the front lens surface and s_2 is the sag of the rear lens surface. Note that in Figure 2.3 the meniscus lens has sags that are both positive, even though the rear surface is negative. In the case of the lens with the concave front surface, this gives a negative sag, since the sign convention requires that sags are measured from the surface to the chord.

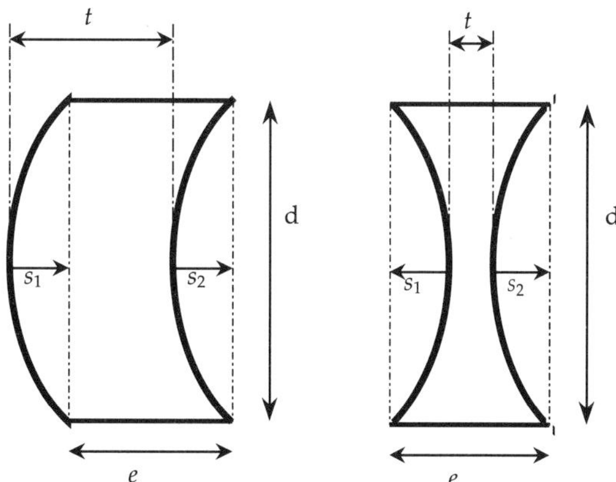

Figure 2.3. Relationship between centre thickness (t), edge thickness (e) and surface sag (s). Sag is measured *from* the lens surface *to* the chord. According to sign convention, distances measured in this way from left to right are positive, while those measured from right to left are negative. The diameter of the lens (d) is equal to $2y$.

Table 2.1 Calculation of edge thickness and centre thickness for spherical lenses

Lens thickness		*Example 1*	*Example 2*	*Example 3*	*Example 4*
To find edge thickness					
Front surface power (D)	F_1	6.00	8.00	1.00	8.00
Rear surface power (D)	F_2	-3.00	-1.00	-10.00	-1.00
Refractive index	n	1.50	1.50	1.50	1.50
Centre thickness (mm)	t	5.00	9.50	1.00	6.00
Lens diameter (mm)	d	65.00	70.00	70.00	70.00
Semi-chord length (mm)	y	32.50	35.00	35.00	35.00
Front surface radius (mm)	$r_1 = 1000(n-1)/F_1$	83.33	62.50	500.00	62.50
Rear surface radius (mm)	$r_2 = 1000(1-n)/F_2$	166.67	500.00	50.00	500.00
Front surface sag (mm)	$s_1 = r_1 - (r_1^2 - y^2)^{1/2}$	6.60	10.72	1.23	10.72
Rear surface sag (mm)	$s_2 = r_2 - (r_2^2 - y^2)^{1/2}$	3.20	1.23	14.29	1.23
Edge thickness (mm)	$e = t - s_1 + s_2$	**1.60**	**0.01**	**14.07**	**-3.49**
		Example 5	*Example 6*	*Example 7*	*Example 8*
To find centre thickness					
Front surface power (D)	F_1	6.00	8.00	1.00	0.50
Rear surface power (D)	F_2	-3.00	-1.00	-10.00	-7.00
Refractive index	n	1.50	1.50	1.50	1.50
Edge thickness (mm)	e	1.00	2.00	14.00	6.00
Lens diameter (mm)	d	65.00	70.00	70.00	70.00
Semi-chord length (mm)	y	32.50	35.00	35.00	35.00
Front surface radius (mm)	$r_1 = 1000(n-1)/F_1$	83.33	62.50	500.00	1000.00
Rear surface radius (mm)	$r_2 = 1000(1-n)/F_2$	166.67	500.00	50.00	71.43
Front surface sag (mm)	$s_1 = r_1 - (r_1^2 - y^2)^{1/2}$	6.60	10.72	1.23	0.61
Rear surface sag (mm)	$s_2 = r_2 - (r_2^2 - y^2)^{1/2}$	3.20	1.23	14.29	9.16
Centre thickness (mm)	$t = e + s_1 - s_2$	**4.40**	**11.49**	**0.93**	**-2.55**

In Table 2.1 it will be noted that Example 4 has a negative edge thickness, and Example 8 a negative centre thickness. What do these values mean? The explanation is shown in Figure 2.4, where a lens is shown with two diameters, d_1 and d_2. Because the centre thickness is too small, an attempt to calculate the edge thickness at a diameter of d_2 would result in a negative edge thickness, as the surfaces have overlapped. The maximum diameter that could be manufactured (for this centre thickness) is d_1, which would give a knife-edged lens. Thus to summarize, if a calculation yields a negative edge or centre thickness, then the lens cannot be manufactured in that form.

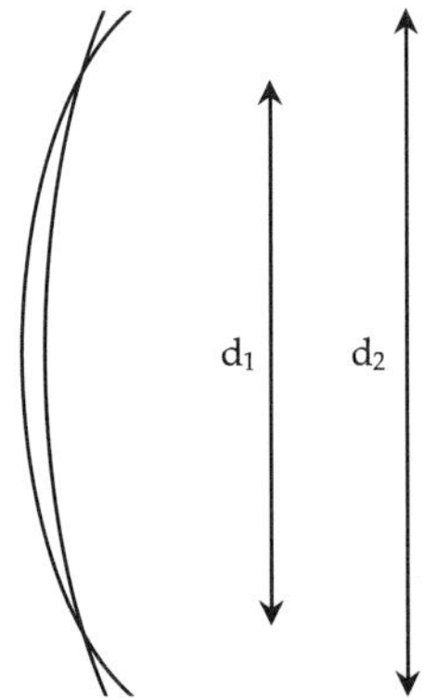

Figure 2.4. The figure shows a meniscus lens with a small centre thickness. The maximum diameter that this lens could be manufactured in is shown by d_1. If the edge thickness for this lens for a diameter of d_2 is calculated, a negative value will be obtained (see Example 4 in Table 2.1) since the surfaces have overlapped. Such a lens could not be manufactured.

Curve variation factor

If a lens sag is known for a given refractive index, it can be useful to know what the sag would be for a different refractive index, for example when predicting the reduction in lens thickness by changing materials. For a given refractive index n_g, and a standard index n_s, the *curve variation factor* is given by:

$$\text{CVF} = (n_s - 1)/(n_g - 1) \qquad \textit{Equation 2.06}$$

The standard value for n_s is 1.523, the refractive index of crown glass. Thus for a material of refractive index 1.700, the CVF would be 0.747. Therefore, if we take as an example a 5.00 D curve with a diameter of 50 mm, the 1.523 material would have a sag of 3.03 mm. Using a 1.700 material for the same curve would give a sag of 2.25 mm using the exact sag formula. However, a quicker method is to multiply the sag for the 1.523 material by the CVF for the 1.700 index, which in this example gives a sag of 2.26 mm.

Magnification of lenses

One factor that will vary with lens form is the magnification experienced by the wearer. *Spectacle magnification* (SM) is defined as the ratio of image size in an eye corrected by a spectacle lens to the image size in the uncorrected eye. In Figure 2.5, a distant object subtends an angle of size w at the principal point of the uncorrected eye, and the image subtends an angle of w' in the corrected eye. Thus:

$$PF = w'/w$$

$$PF = (f' - d)/f'$$

$$PF = 1/(1 - dF') \qquad \textit{Equation 2.07}$$

Equation 2.6 gives the *power factor* (PF) of spectacle magnification. SM can be reduced by making the distance d smaller. This is achieved either by using contact lenses or, for the nearest approach to unity, by using an intraocular lens.

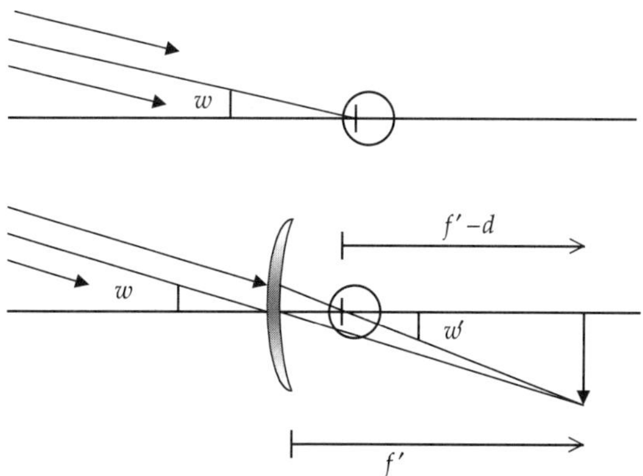

Figure 2.5. Determination of the power factor of spectacle magnification, defined as the ratio of image size in an eye corrected by a spectacle lens to that in an uncorrected eye.

The value of SM is also influenced by the form of the spectacle lens. The discussion above assumes that the lens is optically 'thin'. In the case of a lens with finite thickness, other factors need to be taken into account. In Figure 2.6, a 'thick' lens is shown having back vertex focal length of f'_v and an equivalent focal length of f_e. A thin lens would only have one focal length, as thickness, form, and refractive index are not taken into account. As a meniscus lens is made steeper in form, the equivalent focal length becomes larger in relation to the back vertex focal length, so that the second principal plane may be outside the lens, as shown in Figure 2.6. This increases the magnification, giving rise to the *shape factor* of spectacle magnification (SF). Thus:

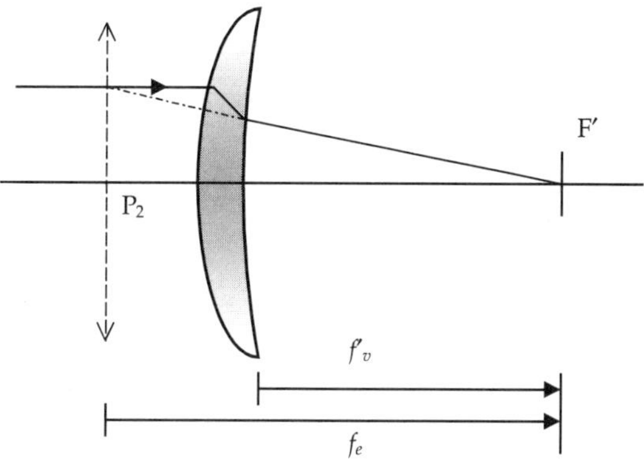

Figure 2.6. The back vertex power of a thick lens (F'_v) is not the same as its equivalent power (Fe), and the second principal plane of the lens (P_2) may lie outside the lens. This gives rise to the shape factor of spectacle magnification.

$$SF = f_e/f'_v = F'_v/F_e$$

Using Equations 1.14 and 1.07:

$$SF = \frac{(F_1 + F_2 - {}^t/_n F_1F_2)/(1 - {}^t/_n F_1)}{(F_1 + F_2 - {}^t/_n F_1F_2)}$$

$$SF = 1/(1 - [t/n]F_1) \qquad \textit{Equation 2.08}$$

In a practical spectacle lens, the total value of spectacle magnification is the product of the shape and power components, thus:

$$SM = PF \times SF \qquad \textit{Equation 2.09}$$

Table 2.2 Calculation of spectacle magnification

Lens thickness		*Example 1*	*Example 2*	*Example 3*	*Example 4*
Spectacle magnification					
Front surface power (D)	F_1	6.00	0.00	2.00	13.00
Rear surface power (D)	F_2	−2.00	4.11	2.10	−2.15
Refractive index	n	1.60	1.60	1.60	1.60
Centre thickness (mm)	t	5.00	5.00	5.00	10.00
Distance to eye (mm)	d	14.00	14.00	14.00	14.00
Back vertex power (D)	F'_v	4.11	4.11	4.11	12.00
Power factor	$PF = 1/(1 - [d/1000]F'_v)$	1.06	1.06	1.06	1.20
Shape factor	$SF = 1/(1 - [t/1000/n]F_1)$	1.02	1.00	1.01	1.09
Spectacle magnification	$SM = PF \times SF$	1.08	1.06	1.07	1.31
(expressed as a percentage)	$SM = 100(SM - 1)$	8.14	6.11	6.78	30.82
		Example 5	*Example 6*	*Example 7*	*Example 8*
Front surface power (D)	F_1	1.00	0.00	−2.00	1.00
Rear surface power (D)	F_2	−5.00	−4.00	−2.00	−21.00
Refractive index	n	1.60	1.60	1.60	1.60
Centre thickness (mm)	t	2.00	2.00	2.00	1.00
Distance to eye (mm)	d	14.00	14.00	14.00	14.00
Back vertex power (D)	F'_v	−4.00	−4.00	−4.00	−20.00
Power factor	$PF = 1/(1 - [d/1000]F'_v)$	0.95	0.95	0.95	0.78
Shape factor	$SF = 1/(1 - [t/1000/n]F_1)$	1.00	1.00	1.00	1.00
Spectacle magnification	$SM = PF \times SF$	0.95	0.95	0.94	0.78
(expressed as a percentage)	$SM = 100(SM - 1)$	−5.18	−5.30	−5.53	−21.83

Some examples of calculations on SM are shown in Table 2.2. Examples 1–3 are positive lenses, all having the same back vertex power of +4.11 D. Note that as the front surface steepens, the overall value of SM increases. As would be expected, the shape factor is unity when the front surface is plane (Example 2). In the case of negative power lenses, the value of SM changes much less with lens form, as a result of the shallower front surfaces used in practical lenses, together with the lower values of centre thickness.

Spectacle magnification problems occur for two main reasons. First there is the case of anisometropia, where one eye has a very small prescription, and the other eye an appreciable ametropia. The problem here is that the image size in the corrected ametopic eye may be so different in size to the other eye that binocular fusion is not possible. The typical example of this is the unilateral aphakic, where both eyes were previously emmetropic. After surgery and correction with spectacles, the aphakic eye will have a spectacle lens power in the order of +12.00 D. As shown in Example 4, this will increase the spectacle magnification to over 30 per cent in the particular lens form illustrated here. In order to maintain binocular vision, the only practical solutions are to try and reduce the distance *d* as much as possible, either by using a contact lens or, even better, by means of an intra-ocular lens.

The second problem that can arise is that when an ametrope is newly corrected the apparent size of familiar objects may change. This again can be of benefit, particularly for myopes. As shown in Example 8, a high myope has a decrease in corrected image size of 21.83 per cent compared with the uncorrected case. Thus although the corrected image will be sharp, it will also be very small, and this can affect the visual acuity. Example 8 shows that this is all due to the power factor, as the shape factor is unity. The only practical way to increase the power factor is to decrease *d* significantly, by using a contact lens.

Lenses for aniseikonia

Lenses with specific (small) values of magnification are known as *iseikonic*, or sometimes as *size* lenses. Specific values of magnification, typically between 2 per cent and 10 per cent,

Table 2.3 Afocal iseikonic lens calculation

Iseikonic lens		
Front surface power (D)	F_1	9.00
Rear surface power (D)	F_2	–9.50
Refractive index	n	1.70
Centre thickness (mm)	t	10.00
Distance to eye (mm)	d	14.00
Back vertex power (D)	F'_v	0.00
Power factor	$PF = 1/(1-[d/1000]F'_v)$	1.00
Shape factor	$SF = 1/(1-[t/1000/n]F_1)$	1.06
Spectacle magnification	$SM = PF \times SF$	1.06
(expressed as a percentage)	$SM = 100(SM - 1)$	5.59

are occasionally used to overcome the binocular vision defect known as aniseikonia.

From Table 2.3 it will be apparent that for a plano lens with significant magnification (6 per cent), lenses with steep surfaces and considerable centre thickness must be used. The heavy weight and poor cosmetic appearance of such lenses means that very few are worn in prescription form. Lenses are also used with high magnifications (200 per cent and more) as low vision aids.

Field of view

There are two approaches to calculating the field of view through a spectacle lens. The first considers the eye in the primary position, with the visual axis coincident with the optical axis of the lens (Figure 2.7a). Here a limiting ray through the nodal point makes an angle a with the axis, and will be imaged in the peripheral retina, but the actual semi-angular field is a', the projected incident ray. As the pupil is close to the nodal point, it does not influence the field of view, but acts as the *aperture stop* of the system.

Secondly, consider an eye rotating to view the limiting ray seen through the edge of the lens with foveal vision. Since the centre of rotation is behind the nodal point (Figure 2.7b), the angle of eye rotation b is less than

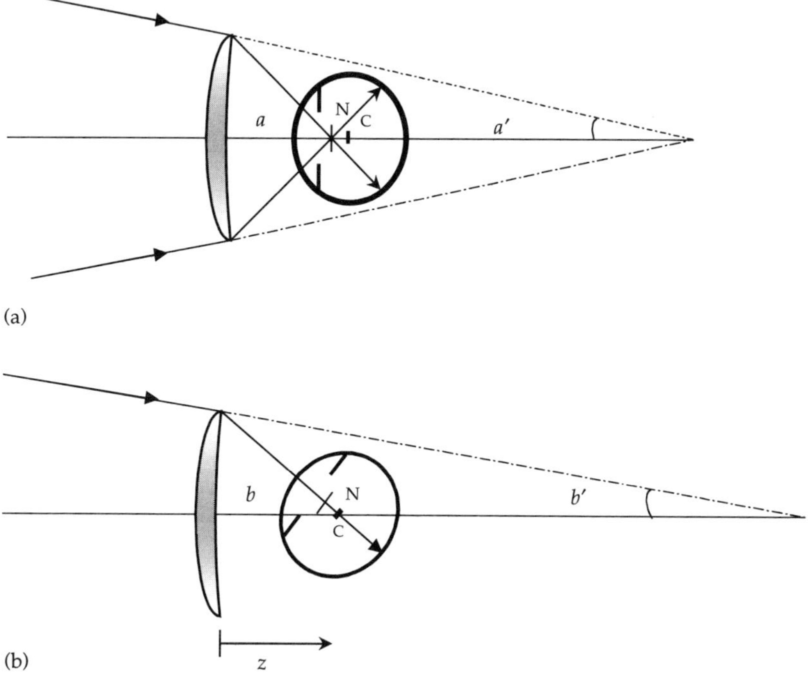

Figure 2.7. Field of view through a positive spectacle lens. (a) The field of view with fixation in the primary position (straight ahead) is considered. The limiting ray through the edge of the lens and the nodal point of the eye (N) makes an angle a with the visual axis, and the projected semi-angular field is a'. (b) The field of view when the eye rotates to look through the edge of the lens is considered. Since the centre of rotation of the eye (C) is behind the nodal point, angle b is smaller than angle a, and the projected semi-angular field b' is also smaller.

the angle a, and the semi-angular field of view b' is smaller than a'.

From Figure 2.7 it can be seen that the controlling factors for the field of view through the lens are:

- Lens prescription, and hence prism at edge of lens
- Lens diameter
- Distance of lens from eye.

The lens acts as the *field stop* for the eye plus lens system. If there is a spectacle frame rim projecting beyond the edge of the spectacle lens, that will obviously also have an effect on the field of view.

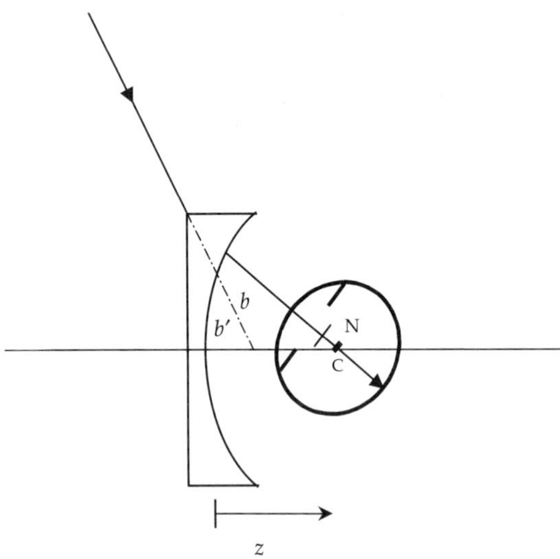

Figure 2.8. Field of view through a negative spectacle lens. The semi-angular field (b') is much larger than for a positive lens (Figure 2.7).

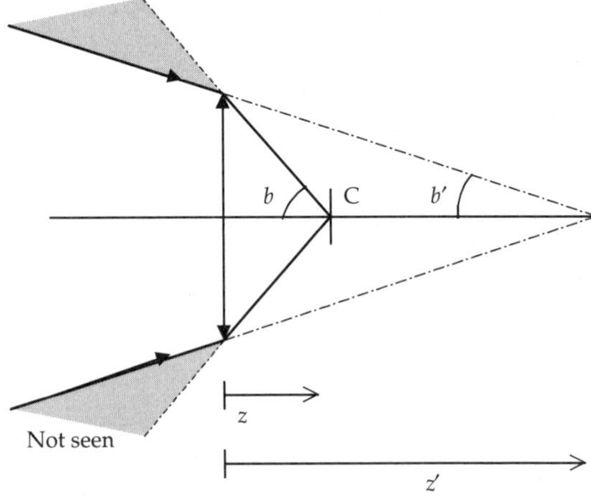

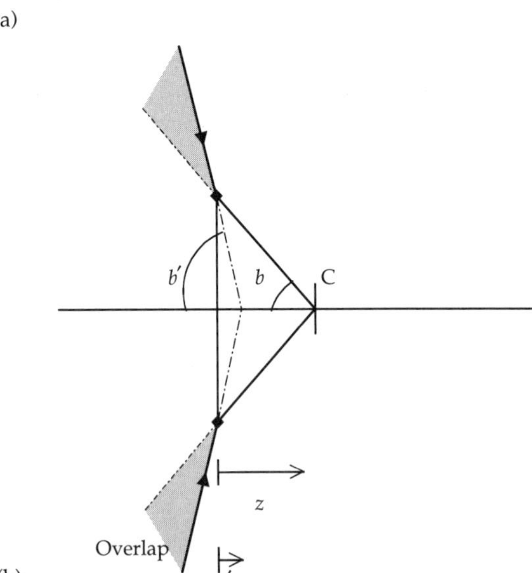

Figure 2.9. (a) Field of view in a positive lens and (b) in a negative lens. In (a), a ring scotoma exists (shaded area) between the clear field visible through the positive lens and the blurred field beyond the lens edge. No such scotoma exists with a negative lens (b), and in fact the fields of view overlap somewhat.

In Figure 2.8 a negative lens is shown, with the reverse effect to that of the plus lens in Figure 2.7. Here, the lens increases the foveal field of view through the spectacle frame aperture compared with a positive power lens or a plano. The consequence of the increased lens power is thus a change in the field of view experienced by the lens wearer. As shown in Figure 2.9, there will be an annular blind area around the periphery of a positive lens where objects cannot be seen either clearly through the lens, or blurred past the edge, unless a head movement is made. This annular blind area is sometimes known as a *roving ring scotoma*. Conversely, a minus lens will produce overlapping visual fields when the eye rotates past the edge of the lens. Thus in a high hypermetrope, the thickness of a spectacle frame rim should be kept as thin as possible in order to maximize the visual field, but rim thickness is less critical for high myopes.

Field of view can be calculated to a first approximation by the method shown in Table 2.4. If the centre of rotation of the eye is considered to be at C, distance z from the

Table 2.4 Calculation of field of view through spectacle lens

Field of view		*Example 1*	*Example 2*	*Example 3*
Lens power (D)	F	20.00	−20.00	0.25
Lens focal length (mm)	f'	50.00	−50.00	4000.00
Centre of rotation distance (mm)	z	−25.00	−25.00	−25.00
Lens diameter (mm)	d	60.00	60.00	60.00
Lens semi–diameter (mm)	$y = d/2$	30.00	30.00	30.00
Reciprocal CR distance (m^{-1})	$Z = 1000/z$	−40.00	−40.00	−40.00
Apparent CR distance (m^{-1})	$Z' = Z + F$	−20.00	−60.00	−39.75
Apparent CR distance (mm)	$z' = 1000/Z'$	−50.00	−16.67	−25.16
Semi–angle of eye rotation (°)	$b = \tan^{-1}(y/z)$	50.19	50.19	50.19
Semi–angle field of view (°)	$b' = \tan^{-1}(y/z')$	30.96	60.95	50.02

spectacle lens, then the lens will image this point at a distance z'. A simple trigonometric calculation will then give the semi-angular field b'. Note that this assumes that the lens is not exhibiting any distortion (see Chapter 7).

Near vision effectivity

In all the discussions thus far it is assumed that a distant object is being imaged by a spectacle lens. In such cases, assuming that the back vertex power is the same in all cases, then all the images will be produced in the same position, at the second principal focus. This is irrespective of the form or material of the lens.

However, when a near object at a finite distance from a lens is viewed, the situation is more complex. In such cases the image position depends not only on the back vertex power of the lens, but also on the form and material. These effects can be calculated either by using a 'step along' calculation method, or alternatively by use of a modified version of the back vertex power formula (Equation 1.07). Table 2.5 illustrates some examples of these calculations for a variety of lens forms, with the object on the lens axis at a distance of 25 cm from the lens. All the

Table 2.5 Exit vergence from a spectacle lens of back vertex power +10.00 D viewing an object 25 cm away on the lens axis. The exit vergence can be seen to vary according to the form of the lens: A, plano–convex; B, biconvex; C, shallow meniscus; D, shallow meniscus; E, Deep meniscus (diagrams not to scale)

Near vision effectivity		*Trial lens A*	*Trial lens B*	*Spectacle lens C*	*Spectacle lens D*	*Spectacle lens E*
Incident vergence	L_1	−4.00	−4.00	−4.00	−4.00	−4.00
Front surface power	F_1	0.00	5.00	10.00	10.00	12.00
Lens thickness	t	0.004	0.005	0.01	0.007	0.012
Rear surface power	F_2	10.00	4.92	−0.71	−0.44	−3.27
Refractive index	n	1.50	1.50	1.50	1.67	1.50
Lens BVP	$F'_v = F_1/(1 - {}^t/_n F_1) + F_2$	10.00	10.00	10.00	10.00	10.00
Input vergence	$L_1 + F_1$	−4.00	1.00	6.00	6.00	8.00
Exit vergence	$L'_2 = (L_1 + F_1)/(1 - {}^t/_n[L_1 + F_1]) + F_2$	6.04	5.92	5.54	5.72	5.27

Incident light

Table 2.6 Exit vergence from a spectacle lens of back vertex power −10.00 D viewing an object 25 cm away on the lens axis. The exit vergence is not crucially dependent on the lens form: A, plano–concave; B, biconcave; C, deep meniscus; D, shallow meniscus (diagrams not to scale)

Near vision effectivity		*Trial lens A*	*Trial lens B*	*Spectacle lens C*	*Spectacle lens D*
Incident vergence	L_1	−4.00	−4.00	−4.00	−4.00
Front surface power	F_1	0.00	−5.00	2.00	1.00
Lens thickness	t	0.002	0.002	0.002	0.002
Rear surface power	F_2	−10.00	−5.03	−12.01	−11.00
Refractive index	n	1.50	1.50	1.50	1.67
Lens BVP	$F'_v = F_1/(1 - {}^t/_n F_1) + F_2$	−10.00	−10.00	−10.00	−10.00
Input vergence	$L_1 + F_1$	−4.00	−9.00	−2.00	−3.00
Exit vergence	$L'_2 = (L_1 + F_2)/(1 - {}^t/_n[L_1 + F_1]) + F_2$	−13.98	−13.92	−14.00	−13.99

Incident light

lenses are of +10.00 D back vertex power, but the form varies considerable. Lens A is a plano-convex trial case lens, manufactured so that the rear surface is curved. This lens form has the advantage that the BVP does not alter with lens thickness. It will be noted from the value of exit vergence (L'_2) that the value does not depart significantly from the theoretical 'thin' lens value of +6.00. The same is true for the second type of trial case lens (B), which is biconvex in form. However, note the situation in the three spectacle lens forms illustrated. Lens C is a shallow meniscus lens, of normal (1.50) refractive index. The exit vergence of +5.54 is approximately half a dioptre less than the trial lens value. This means that the spectacle lens will be giving an effective near power that is undercorrected by half a dioptre. The situation is improved in lens D, which is a thinner, flatter, high-index meniscus; however, the lens power is still undercorrected by a quarter of a dioptre. The final lens (E) is a steep meniscus form, and illustrates that the effect of a deeply curved front surface and appreciable centre thickness is to give a near error of three-quarters of a dioptre. How much of a problem this effect causes depends on what happens to the lens power at other points on the lens, as described in Chapter 7.

In the case of negative power lenses, there is much less difference between the trial case lens exit vergence and that from the finished spectacle lens, as shown in Table 2.6. This is because minus lenses have much flatter front surface curves than is the case with plus powers, and also the centre thicknesses are less.

Summary

In this chapter, the effects of lens form on spherical powered lenses have been considered. Lens form can affect the thickness, magnification and field of view through a lens, and also the effectivity for viewing near objects.

Formulae

Formula	*Name*	*Equation number*
$s = r - \sqrt{(r^2 - y^2)}$	Exact sag formula for sag	2.01
$r = (y^2 + s^2)/(2s)$	Exact sag formula for radius	2.02
$s = y^2/(2r)$	Approximate sag formula for sag	2.03
$r = y^2/(2s)$	Approximate sag formula for radius	2.04
$e = t - s_1 + s_2$	Edge thickness	2.05
$\text{CVF} = (n_s - 1)/(n_g - 1)$	Curve variation factor	2.06
$\text{PF} = 1/(1 - dF')$	Power factor of spectacle magnification	2.07
$\text{SF} = 1/(1 - (^t/_n)F_1)$	Shape factor of spectacle magnification	2.08
$\text{SM} = \text{PF} \times \text{SF}$	Spectacle magnification	2.09

Exercises

Questions

1. Using thin lens approximations, all of the following lenses have the same power of +6.00 DS. What are the front and back vertex powers of each lens if the centre thickness is 4 mm and the refractive index of the material is 1.5?

	F1	*F2*
a.	+3.00	+3.00
b.	+1.00	+5.00
c.	plano	+6.00
d.	+10.00	–4.00
e.	+8.25	–2.25

   Given these values, why do you consider that full aperture trial lenses are made in the biconvex/biconcave form?
2. What is the sag of a surface that has a diameter of 50 mm, a surface power of +8 D and is made of 1.6 index glass?
3. A lens surface has a sag of 1.7 mm across its 45 mm diameter. The lens is made of 1.6 index plastics. What is the radius of curvature of the surface?
4. A lens has a surface power of +10 D. The sag of the surface is 10 mm and the refractive index of the lens is 1.5. What is the diameter of the lens?
5. A lens is made of crown glass ($n = 1.523$) and has a diameter of 48 mm. The power of the surface is +10 D. By how much is the answer in error if the sag of the surface is calculated by the approximate sag formula rather than by using the exact sag formula?
6. A negative lens is made with a front surface power of +2 D and a rear surface power of –7 D. The lens has a centre thickness of 1 mm and is a round lens of diameter 60 mm. What is the edge thickness if the lens is made of 1.5 index material? How much thinner is the lens at the edge if a high index material ($n = 1.8$) is used instead?
7. A plano-convex lens is made with a front surface power of +6 D of a 1.5 index material. What will the centre thickness be if the lens is to be made knife-edge with a diameter of 60 mm?
8. What is the centre thickness of a lens that has a front surface power of +12.25 D and a rear surface power of –4.00 D if the edge thickness of the 46 mm diameter lens is 1 mm and the refractive index of the lens material is 1.491? The diameter of the lens required is increased to 70 mm. What is the new centre thickness?
9. A myopic spectacle wearer wears a lens with a front surface power of +2 D and a back surface power of –10 D. The lenses have a centre thickness of 1 mm, a refractive index of 1.5 and the spectacles are worn 14 mm from the eye. What spectacle magnification does the person experience? If the person pushes their spectacles up their nose, giving them a vertex distance of 8 mm, what is the spectacle magnification now?
10. On refraction, a patient is found to require +8.00 D in order to read comfortably at 25 cm. The trial lens used in the refraction is of biconvex form (front surface power +4 D, rear surface power +3.95 D, centre thickness 5 mm, index 1.5). The patient is prescribed this back vertex power in spectacles, which are made up in meniscus form (front surface power +10 D, rear surface power –2.71 D, centre thickness 10 mm, index 1.5). The patient returns complaining of problems with the glasses. What is the difference between the exit vergence required and that provided by the spectacles? What problems is the patient likely to be complaining of?

Answers

1. a. +6.03 DS, +6.03 DS; b. +6.00 DS, +6.07 DS; c. +6.00 DS, +6.10 DS; d. +6.27 DS, +6.04 DS; e. +6.18 DS, +6.01 DS
2. 4.29 mm
3. 150 mm
4. 60 mm
5. 0.32 mm
6. 5.80 mm; 1.92 mm or 33 per cent thinner
7. 5.59 mm
8. 6.09 mm; 16.45 mm
9. 0.901; 0.941
10. +0.41 D

3

Astigmatic lens forms

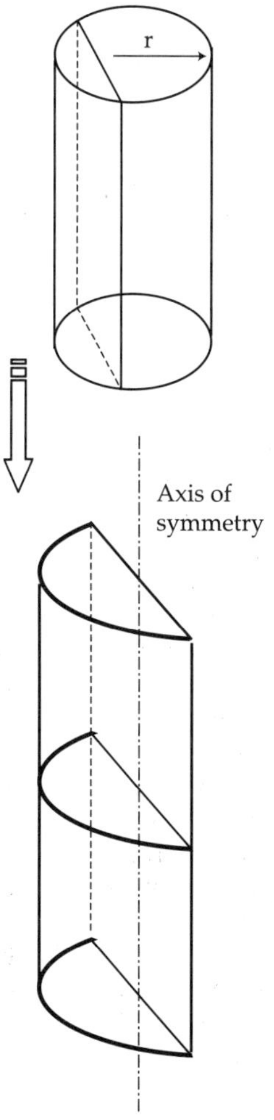

Figure 3.1. The plane positive cylindrical lens can be imagined as being taken as a section of transparent rod.

Introduction

An astigmatic lens or lens system is one that does not produce a point image from a point object. The human eye is very often astigmatic, thus simple spherical lenses cannot always be used to provide a clear image. In order to correct an astigmatic eye, therefore, an astigmatic lens is used to neutralize the power error of the eye.

The simplest astigmatic lens form is the *cylindrical* lens (Figure 3.1). Note that the spherical radius of curvature of the lens is the same for all sections perpendicular to the axis of symmetry, and that along the axis of symmetry the thickness is constant. Cylindrical lenses can also be produced in negative form (Figure 3.2).

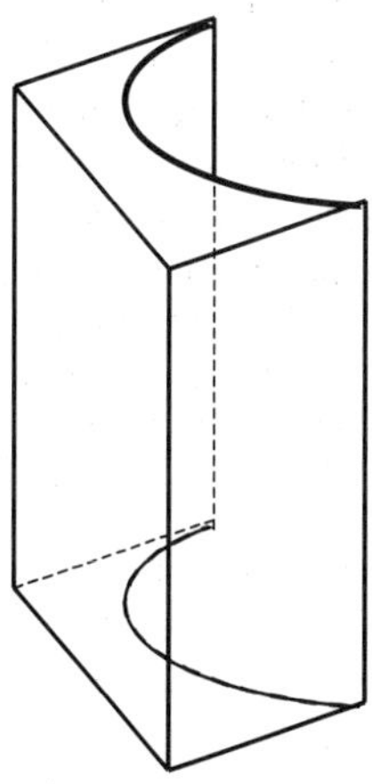

Figure 3.2. A plane negative cylindrical lens.

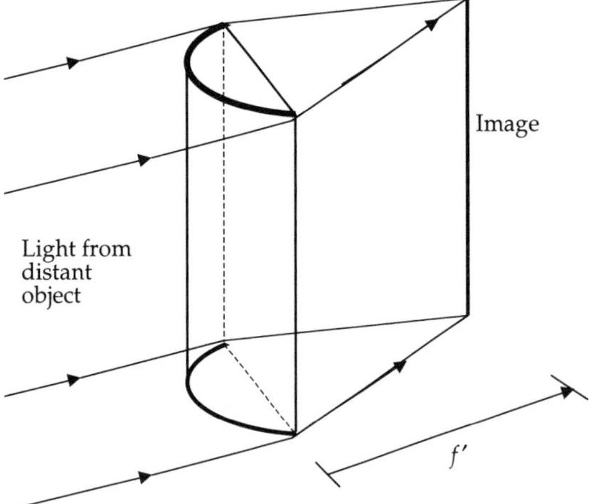

Figure 3.3. Image formation of cylindrical lens parallel to axis of symmetry.

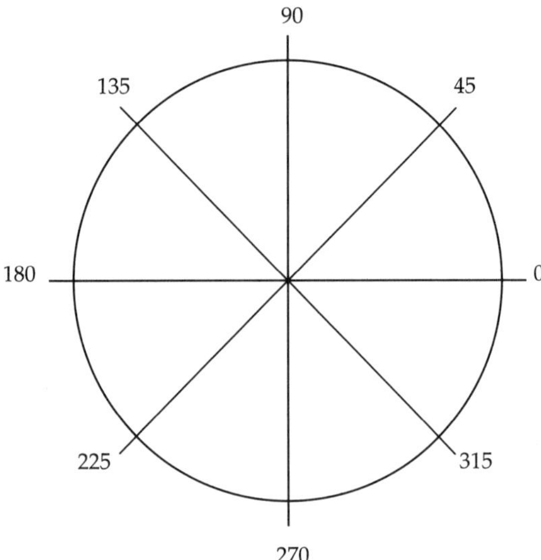

Figure 3.4. Standard axis notation when viewing the front surface of a lens (BS EN ISO 8429, 1997).

A cylindrical lens will produce a *line* image from a point object (Figure 3.3), the line being parallel to the axis of symmetry. Object and image positions can be found by using the same equations as for spherical surfaces and lenses (Chapter 1).

Although plane cylindrical lenses as described can be used in spectacles, it is more common to use a cylindrical surface in combination with a spherical surface, in order to provide a *sphero-cylindrical* lens.

Notation for cylindrical lenses

A lens with purely cylindrical power would be described as, for example, –6.00 DC (dioptres cylindrical) in order to differentiate from the spherical case, which would be described as –6.00 DS (dioptres spherical).

Because cylindrical surfaces are not rotationally symmetrical about the midpoint, a notation is required for their positioning in front of the eye. This is achieved by specifying the angle between the axis of symmetry of the cylinder (which is always simply referred to as the 'axis') and the horizontal. The universally used 'standard' axis notation (BS EN ISO 8429, 1997) uses a protractor that reads anticlockwise when looking at the face of a lens wearer (Figure 3.4). Angles up to 180° are used for the axes of cylinders, the full 360° protractor only being required for the base direction of prisms (Chapter 4). When describing a horizontal cylinder axis, it is conventional to use the angle 180, rather than zero. Note that degree signs are not used when writing the specification of cylinder axes.

Radii of cylindrical surfaces

From Figure 3.1 it should be apparent that the curvature of a cylindrical surface of radius r is at a maximum perpendicular to the axis of symmetry, and a minimum (with infinite radius) parallel to the axis. Thus if a surface of radius +100 mm is worked on material of refractive index 1.5, then the surface power will vary from zero along the axis, to a maximum of $F = 1000(n - 1)/r = 500/100 = +5.00$ D (Equation 1.03). Indeed the maxima and the minima will be the only two powers that can be optically resolved. However, the surface curvature will vary between these maximum and minimum values. In Figure 3.5, a cylindrical surface has a radius of curvature r perpendicular to the cylindrical axis. Consider a section through this surface, at an angle of θ to the axis of symmetry. What will be the radius at a point P on the surface?

An oblique section through a cylinder will be in the shape of an ellipse, where the semi-major axis length is a and the semi-minor b.

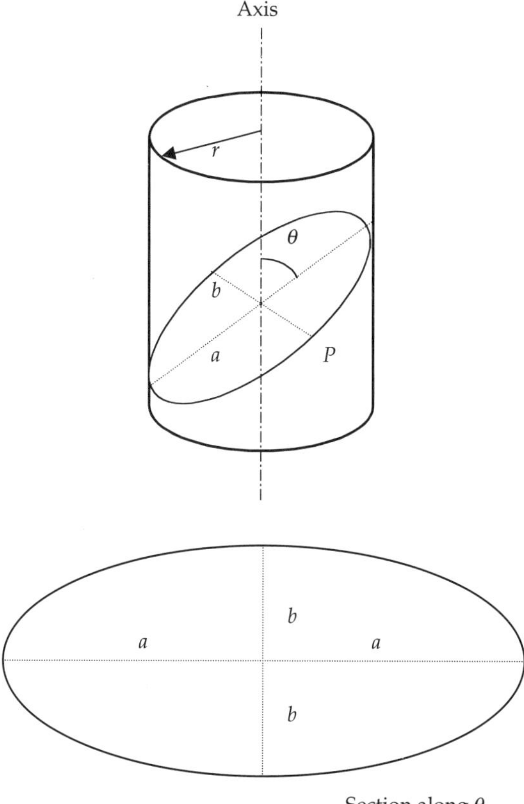

Figure 3.5. Calculation of cylindrical surface curvature at any angle to the axis.

Note that $r = b$. From the geometry of the ellipse, the radius (r_θ) at point P will be:

$$r_\theta = a^2/b = (r/\sin\theta)^2/r = r/\sin^2\theta \quad \textit{Equation 3.01}$$

For example, if a surface has a radius of 100 mm, what will be the radius at 30° to the axis? The sine of 30° is 0.5, thus $r_{30} = 100/(0.5^2) = 100/0.25 = 400$ mm.

If a section is taken parallel to the axis, then $\theta = 0°$, and $\sin\theta = 0$. Thus r_θ will be infinite as the cylinder is plane parallel to the axis. A section perpendicular to the axis will have $\theta = 90°$, $\sin\theta = 1$, and $r_\theta = r$ as you would expect.

A useful application of this result is to demonstrate that any spherical surface can be replaced by two identical plane cylinders, with axes mutually perpendicular. In Figure 3.6, two cylinders with axes 90 and 180 have the same curvature R. A generalized axis θ is taken, along which the curvature is $R\theta$. Since

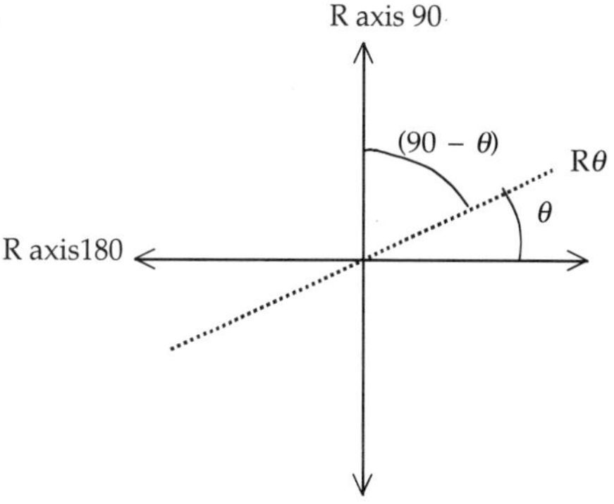

Figure 3.6. Spherical surfaces represented by two cylinders with identical curvature having axes mutually perpendicular.

$R = 1/r$, and the sin of $(90 - \theta) = \cos\theta$, then the curvature along θ due to the two cylinders is:

$$\begin{aligned} R\theta &= R\sin^2\theta + R\cos^2\theta \\ &= R(\sin^2\theta + \cos^2\theta) \\ &= R(1) \\ &= R \end{aligned}$$

Thus, for example, a +3.00 DS surface could be replaced by +3.00 DC × 90 combined with +3.00 DC × 180, or +3.00 DC × 20 combined with +3.00 DC × 110, and so on.

Sags and thicknesses of cylindrical lenses

If the thickness of a cylindrical or sphero-cylindrical lens is required along or perpendicular to the axis of symmetry, then the problem is similar to the spherical lens situation, except that there are two meridians to deal with. For example, consider the lens with surface powers +3.00 DS and +2.00 DC axis 90. If the lens is 60 mm round, the refractive index is 1.5 and the minimum edge thickness is 2.0 mm, what will be the centre thickness and maximum edge thickness?

The calculation method is shown in Table 3.1 using the sag formulae defined in Chapter 2, and a schematic diagram of sections through the lens is shown in Figure 3.7. Note in particular that the rear surface radius is negative, despite the surface power being positive, and this gives a negative sag. The

Table 3.1 Maximum and minimum edge thicknesses of sphero–cylindrical lenses

Lens refractive index	n	1.50
Minimum edge thickness (mm)	e_{min}	2.00
Power of front surface (D)	F_1	3.00
Power of rear surface (D)	F_2	2.00
Lens diameter (mm)	d	60.00
Radius of front surface (mm)	$r_1 = 1000(n-1)/F_1$	166.67
Radius of rear surface (mm)	$r_2 = 1000(1-n)/F_2$	–250.00
Semi–chord length (mm)	$y = d/2$	30.00
Sag of front surface (mm)	$s_1 = r_1 - (r_1^2 - y^2)^{0.5}$	2.72
Sag of rear surface (mm)	$s_2 = r_2 + (r_2^2 - y^2)^{0.5}$	–1.81
Centre thickness (mm)	$t = e_{min} + s_1 - s_2$	6.53
Maximum edge thickness (mm)	$e_{max} = t - s_1$	3.81

maximum edge thickness will be along 90, as this is the direction where the rear surface convex cylinder has zero sag.

Let us consider a second example, where the cylinder power is negative, and we need to know not only the minimum edge thickness having been given the maximum, but also the edge thickness along the horizontal meridian. The lens surface powers are +1.00 DS on the front surface and the rear surface is –6.00 DC axis 160. Thus along the horizontal meridian the cylinder has a relative axis (θ) of 20°.

Note that the edge thickness along 180 is close to the minimum value, as the cylinder axis is only 20° relative to the horizontal.

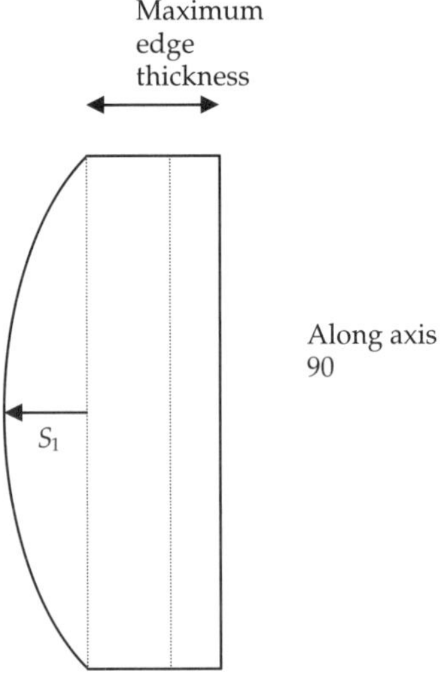

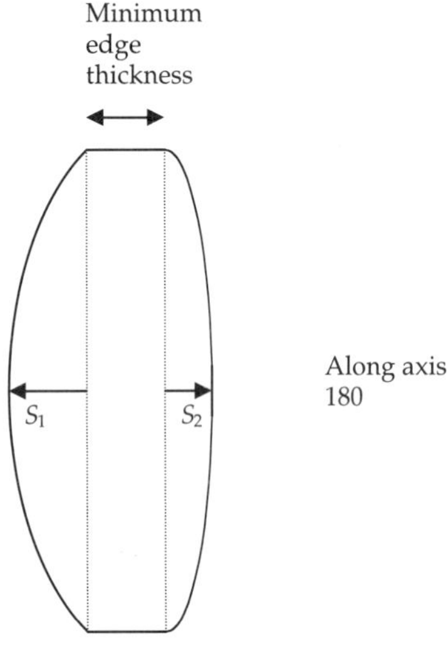

Figure 3.7. Edge thickness of a sphero-cylindrical lens along its axis and perpendicular to the axis. The spherical power is shown as being on the front surface of the lens and the cylindrical power on the rear surface.

Combination of cylindrical lenses

As mentioned above, sphero-cylindrical lens combinations are common in ophthalmic optics. Such lenses can be made in alternative forms. Consider the example of a +3.00 DS front surface combined with a +2.00 DC axis 90 to give a thin lens. This is conventionally written as +3.00 DS/+2.00 DC × 90, or +3.00/+2.00 × 90.

For analytical purposes, it can be useful to write this in terms of purely cylindrical powers. Thus we have already shown that the +3.00 DS can be replaced by +3.00 DC × 90 combined with +3.00 DC × 180. If we now add in the +2.00 DC × 90, the total effect is +5.00 DC × 90/+3.00 DC × 180. Note that the '/' symbol indicates 'combined with'. This notation is known as the *cross-cylinder* form, and is useful for analytical purposes.

What would happen if the combination +5.00 DS/–2.00 DC × 180 were considered? Here the sphere would be represented by +5.00 DC × 90/+5.00 DC × 180. Adding in the cylinder gives +5.00 DC × 90/+3.00 DC × 180, the same result as achieved before. Thus there are two alternative sphero-cylindrical forms, and these can be exchanged by a process of transposition.

Table 3.2 Edge thickness of sphero–cylindrical lens at specified point

Minimum edge thickness (mm)	e_{min}	5.00
Power of front surface (D)	F_1	1.00
Power of rear surface (D)	F_2	–6.00
Lens diameter (mm)	d	50.00
Radius of front surface (mm)	$r_1 = 1000(n-1)/F_1$	500.00
Radius of rear surface (mm)	$r_2 = 1000(1-n)/F_2$	83.33
Semi–chord length (mm)	$y = d/2$	25.00
Sag of front surface (mm)	$s_1 = r_1 - (r_1^2 - y^2)^{0.5}$	0.63
Sag of rear surface (mm)	$s_2 = r_2 - (r_2^2 - y^2)^{0.5}$	3.84
Centre thickness (mm)	$t = e_{min} + s_1$	5.63
Maximum edge thickness (mm)	$e_{max} = t - s_1 + s_2$	8.84
Relative angle (°)	θ	20
	$\sin^2\theta$	0.1170
Effective r_2 along 180 (mm)	$r_{180} = r_2/\sin^2\theta$	712.39
Rear surface sag along 180 (mm)	$s_{2(180)} = r_{2(180)} - (r_{2(180)}^2 - y^2)^{0.5}$	0.44
Edge thickness along 180 (mm)	$e_{180} = t - s_1 + s_{2(180)}$	5.44

Rules for transposition of sphero-cylindrical lenses

1. Add sphere to cylinder to give new spherical power.
2. Change sign of cylinder to give new cylinder.
3. Change axis by 90°. If original cylinder axis is ≤90 then add 90; if original cylinder axis is >90, then subtract 90.

Astigmatic lens forms

Astigmatic lens forms using plane cylinders are described as *flat* lenses. As with spherical forms (see Chapter 2), flat lens forms can suffer from poor optical performance when used for off-axis vision. In order to remedy this problem, *curved* form lenses are used, these requiring a *toroidal* surface to incorporate a cylindrical effect.

Toroidal surfaces have two different finite radii in mutually perpendicular meridians. Perhaps the easiest form to visualize is the so-called *barrel* form. In Figure 3.8 a barrel form toroid is shown with axis of symmetry vertical. Note that a typical lens surface represents only a small area of the barrel surface, and in low power cylinders a toroidal surface can be difficult to distinguish from a spherical surface by inspection. Relative to a point P on the surface, the centre of curvature for a vertical section is C_v, and the centre of curvature of a horizontal (equatorial) section is C_h. In a barrel form C_v is greater than C_h, but in an alternative form, the tyre, C_h is greater than than C_v.

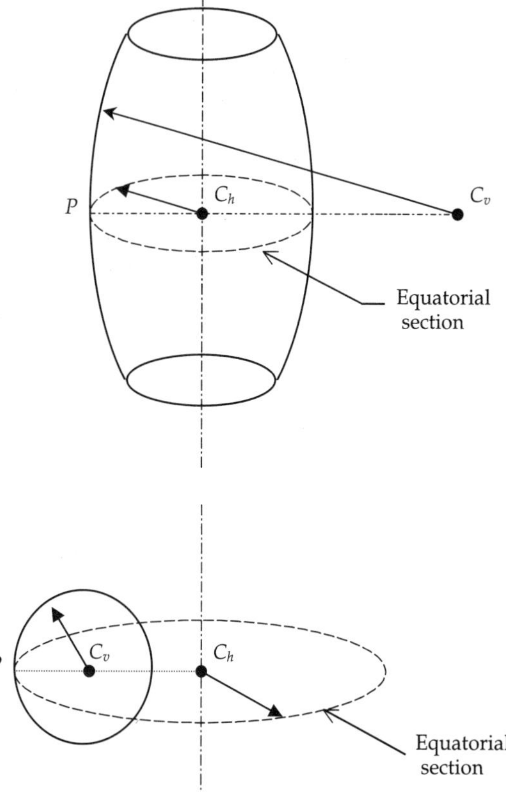

Figure 3.8. Barrel toroidal surface (top) and tyre form (bottom).

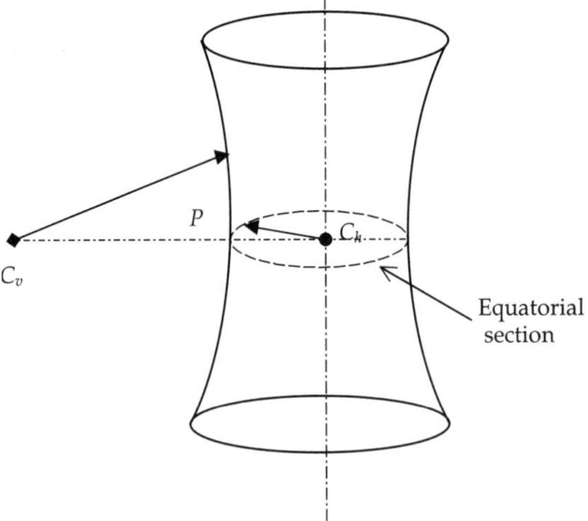

Figure 3.9. Capstan form toroidal surface.

One further type of toroidal surface should be considered, although it is rarely used. This is the capstan form (Figure 3.9). Here the positions of C_v and C_h are on opposite sides of the surface. Hence the two powers on the surface are of opposite sign. Capstan toroidal surfaces have been used in the past on cylindrical aniseikonic lenses (Chapter 2).

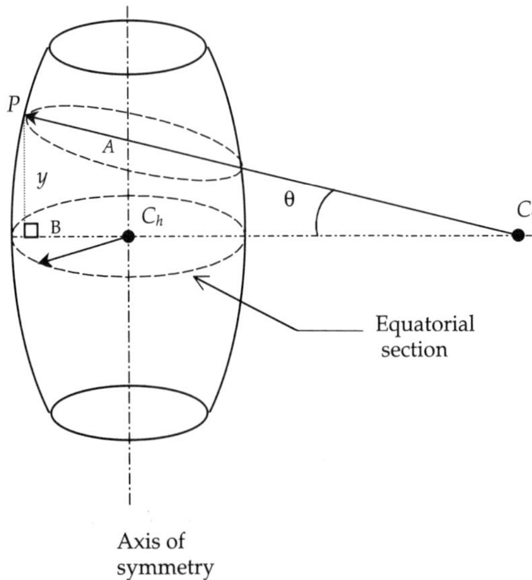

Figure 3.10. Radii of curvature at a non-equatorial point (P) on a toroidal surface. C_v is the centre of curvature of the vertical surface, which has a radius of curvature r_v. C_h is the centre of curvature of the horizontal surface, which has a radius of curvature r_h.

The three forms of toroidal surface have been considered with the point of reference (P) on an equatorial section. But what happens if P is not on the equator? In Figure 3.10, P is at a distance y above the equator of a barrel toroidal surface. The vertical radius (parallel to the axis of symmetry) is unchanged, so that $PC_v = r_v$. But in a horizontal section (perpendicular to the axis of symmetry), the radius (r_h) measured along the normal is now PA. Thus:

$$C_vC_h = (r_v - r_h)$$

$$AC_v = (r_v - r_h)/\cos\theta$$

$$r_\theta = PA = PC_v - AC_v$$

$$r_\theta = r_v - [(r_v - r_h)/\cos\theta] \qquad \textit{Equation 3.02}$$

This has implications in lens manufacture, since a smoothing or polishing tool cannot be made to move randomly over a toroidal surface with closely matching curves.

Toric lenses

A lens with a toroidal surface is known as a *toric* lens. Toric lenses may very occasionally have two toroidal surfaces, for example, in order to make a very high power cylindrical lens, but such items are rare.

Conventionally, a toric lens will have one spherical surface and one toroidal surface. The toroidal surface may be the front or back surface. The specification is commonly written as, for example:

$$\frac{+6.00\text{ DS}}{-3.00\text{ DC} \times 30/-5.00\text{ DC} \times 120}$$

The spherical front surface is written above the line, with the specification of the toroidal rear surface being written beneath. This lens could also have been specified as:

$$\frac{+5.00\text{ DC} \times 120/+7.00\text{ DC} \times 30}{-4.00\text{ DS}}$$

This second example is a front surface toroidal lens, the first being a back surface toroidal lens. Rear surface toroidal lenses are currently the most commonly used form, mainly for reasons of manufacturing convenience. If the lenses are considered to be 'thin', then both the above examples will have the same power.

$$\frac{+5.00\text{ DC} \times 120/+7.00\text{ DC} \times 30}{-4.00\text{ DS}}$$

The first step is to add the first power of the toroidal surface to the spherical power, giving +1.00 × 120. Next, the second power on the toroidal surface is added to the spherical power, giving +3.00 × 30. This is equivalent to a sphero-cylindrical power of +1.00/+2.00 × 30.

$$\frac{+5.00\text{ DC} \times 120/+7.00\text{ DC} \times 30}{-4.00\text{ DS}}$$

Unlike a sphero-cylindrical form of lens, where there are only two alternative specifications, a toric lens can have a virtually infinite variety of forms, depending on the curvature of the spherical surface.

Nomenclature of toric lenses

The traditional nomenclature for a toric lens is:

- Sphere curve: power of the spherical surface
- Base curve: lowest absolute power (longest radius) on the toroidal surface
- Cross curve: highest absolute power (shortest radius) on the toroidal surface.

The terms 'base curve' and 'cross curve' originate from the traditional method of manufacturing front surface toric glass single vision lenses. The term 'base curve' is now more likely to be used to describe the front spherical curve of a semi-finished lens which is designed to have a toroidal surface subsequently placed on the back.

Transposition of toric specifications

Transposition between toric forms can be deduced from the discussion above, but here are the steps for the various transpositions.

Toric to sphero-cylindrical form

1. Add sphere curve of toric to first power of toroidal surface to give first power and axis of cross-cylinder form.
2. Add sphere curve of toric to second power of toroidal surface to give second power and axis of cross-cylinder form.
3. Convert cross-cylinder form to sphero-cylindrical form.

Example:

$$\frac{+3.00\text{ DS}}{-5.00\text{ DC} \times 50/-6.00\text{ DC} \times 140}$$

1. +3.00 DS + (–5.00 DC) × 50 ⇒ –2.00 DC × 50
2. +3.00 DS + (–6.00 DC) × 140 ⇒ –3.00 DC × 140
3. –2.00 DS/–1.00 DC × 140.

Sphero-cylindrical to toric form with specific base curve on toroidal surface

1. Transpose sphero-cylindrical form to the sphero-cylindrical form with the same sign of cylinder as the power of the base curve.
2. Write down base curve with axis 90° to cylinder axis.
3. Cross curve is base curve plus cylinder power with axis the same as cylinder axis.
4. Subtract base curve from sphere of sphero-cylindrical form to give sphere surface of toric.

Example:

+8.00 DS/–3.00 DC × 180, on +9.00 DC toroidal base curve

1. +8.00/–3.00 × 180 ⇒ +5.00/+3.00 × 90
2. +9.00 × 180
3. +9.00 + (+3.00) × 90 ⇒ +12.00 × 90
4. +5.00 – (+9.00) ⇒ –4.00

Finished form:

$$\frac{+9.00 \times 180/+12.00 \times 90}{-4.00}$$

Sphero-cylindrical to toric form with specific spherical surface

1. Convert to cross-cylindrical form.
2. Subtract spherical surface from each power of the cross-cylinder form to give the new powers and associated axes for the toroidal surface.

Example:

–1.00/+2.00 × 165 on +4.00 DS curve

1. –1.00 × 75/+1.00 × 165
2. –1.00 – (+4.00) ⇒ –5.00 × 75 and
   +1.00 – (+4.00) ⇒ –3.00 × 165

Finished form:

$$\frac{+4.00}{-3.00 \times 165/-5.00 \times 75}$$

Table 3.3 Exact transposition of thick toroidal lens forms

Exact transposition		*Example 1*	*Example 2 (axis 180)*	*Example 2 (axis 90)*
Incident vergence (m^{-1})	L_1	−11.00	−16.00	−13.00
First surface power (D)	F_1	−1.00	−3.00	−3.00
Refractive index	n	1.50	1.50	1.50
Lens thickness (m)	t	0.01	0.01	0.01
Input vergence (m^{-1})	$V = L_1 + F_1$	−12.00	−19.00	−16.00
Vergence at second surface (m^{-1})	$L_2 = V/(1 - {}^t/_n V)$	−11.11	−16.86	−14.46
As L'_2 is required to be zero, second surface power (D)	$F_2 = -L_2$	+11.11	+16.86	+14.46

'Exact' transposition

So far we have only considered transposition in relation to thin lenses. However, in practical lens forms we also have to consider the effects of thickness and refractive index. For example, if we have a lens prescription of +8.00/+3.00 × 90, and it is required in toric form, then the thin lens version on, say, a sphere curve of +12.00 DS would be:

$$\frac{+12.00}{-1.00 \times 90/-4.00 \times 180}$$

However, if the lens is of thickness 10 mm, in 1.5 refractive index material, then these surface curves would give a back vertex power of +12.04 × 90/+9.04 × 180, equivalent to a sphero-cylinder form of +9.04/+3.00 × 90. Thus the front surface in this case must be reduced in power (compensated) to give the correct BVP at the required thickness. One way of doing this is shown in Table 3.3. Example 1 considers the 90° axis in the example given above. The calculation is reversed, so that incident light enters the rear concave surface divergent from the second principal focus. After refraction by the first (rear) surface and passing through the required thickness, the vergence incident at the second (front) surface is found (L_2). The power of the second surface is then $-L_2$ so that $L'_2 = 0$ (Figure 3.11). If light from a distant object (incident vergence zero) is then passed through the lens, it will focus at the required back vertex focal length.

Thus the correct specification for the above lens (prescription +8.00/+3.00 × 90, lens thickness 10 mm, and refractive index 1.5) becomes:

$$\frac{+11.11}{-1.00 \times 90/-4.00 \times 180} \quad \text{(Example 1)}$$

The situation is different if a front toroidal surface is required, as in this case both of the front surface powers must be compensated. For example, consider the prescription +13.00/+3.00 × 90, to be made in toric form with a −3.00 D sphere curve, centre thickness 10 mm, refractive index 1.50. The thin lens version of the toric specification would be:

$$\frac{+16.00 \times 180/+19.00 \times 90}{-3.00}$$

However, as shown in Table 3.3, the required powers for an exact specification on a thick lens would be:

$$\frac{+14.46 \times 180/+16.86 \times 90}{-3.00} \quad \text{(Example 2)}$$

Note that in this case the front surface cylindrical difference is 2.40 D, even though the astigmatic difference measured at the rear surface is 3.00 D.

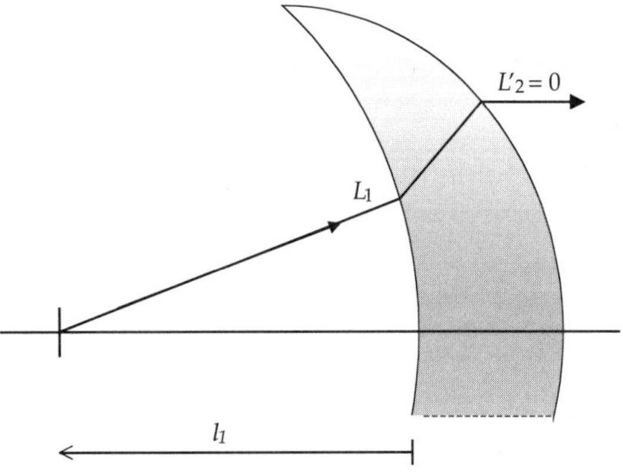

Figure 3.11. Reverse ray trace to find compensated front surface power of a thick toric lens.

Obliquely crossed cylinders

Cylindrical lenses in combination, where the axes are not parallel or mutually perpendicular, are called *obliquely crossed.* Any pair of cylindrical lenses (with associated sphere, if present) can be resolved into a single spherocylindrical combination. Unfortunately, this is somewhat more complex than resolving obliquely crossed prisms (Chapter 4).

We have already shown in this chapter (Equation 3.01) that the effective power at a given angle θ to the axis of a cylinder with power F is $F\sin^2\theta$. Thus along the axis, the power of a cylinder is at a minimum, and is maximum perpendicular to the axis. The effects of combining two plane cylinders are shown in Table 3.4. Here the example of +1.00 × 20 combined with +3.00 × 60 is used to illustrate the power components at 10° intervals, as well as the resultant derived from adding the two together. Note that the resultant has a minimum and maximum value, these being the principal powers of the combination in cross-cylinder form.

Table 3.4 Analysis of obliquely crossed cylinders. Note that the principal meridians of the combined cylinders are different to those for either cylinder individually

Angle	*B*	*C*	*Sum (B + C)*
0	0.12	2.25	2.37
10	0.03	1.76	1.79
20	0.00	1.24	1.24
30	0.03	0.75	0.78
40	0.12	0.35	0.47
50	0.25	0.09	0.34
60	0.41	0.00	0.41
70	0.59	0.09	0.68
80	0.75	0.35	1.10
90	0.88	0.75	1.63
100	0.97	1.24	2.21
110	1.00	1.76	2.76
120	0.97	2.25	3.22
130	0.88	2.65	3.53
140	0.75	2.91	3.66
150	0.59	3.00	3.59
160	0.41	2.91	3.32
170	0.25	2.65	2.90

Column B = 1.00 × sin²(20 – angle);
Column C = 3.00 × sin²2(60 – angle).

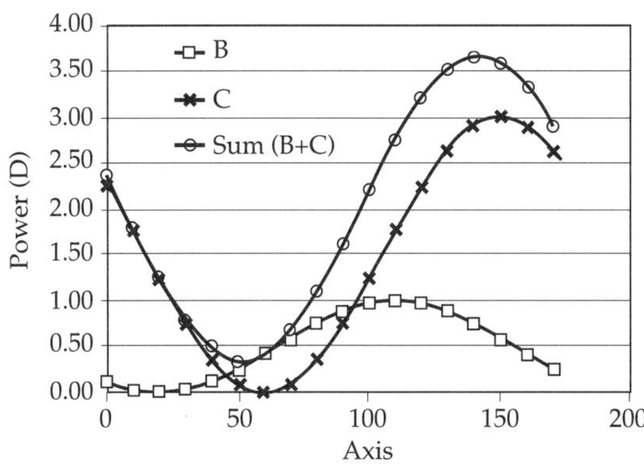

Figure 3.12. Analysis of crossed cylinders.

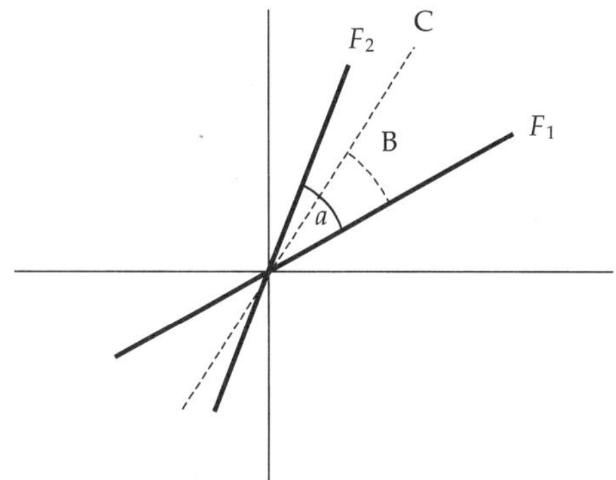

Figure 3.13. Resolution of obliquely crossed cylinders.

Thus it is possible to derive the power of a combination of cylinders by graphical methods, but there is a simpler solution. In Figure 3.13, two cylindrical lenses are shown, F_1 and F_2. Their axes are separated by an angle a. A resultant power component C has an angle of B from the axis of F_1. The effect of the two cylinders F_1 and F_2 at F can be calculated from:

$$F_A = F_1 \sin^2 B + F_2 \sin^2(a - B) \qquad \textit{Equation 3.03}$$

Perpendicular to the axis of C the power is:

$$F_B = F_1 \sin^2 (90 - B) + F_2 \sin^2(90 - a - B)$$

Which can also be written as:

$$F_B = F_1 \cos^2 B + F_2 \cos^2(a - B) \qquad \textit{Equation 3.04}$$

If these two values are the maximum and minimum, then the cylinder power of the resultant sphero-cylinder is:

$$C = F_B - F_A$$

$$C = F_1 \cos^2 B + F_2 \cos^2(a - B) - [F_1 \sin^2 B + F_2 \sin^2(a - B)] \qquad \textit{Equation 3.05}$$

Table 3.5 Calculation of the resultant sphero–cylindrical lens when two cylinders are crossed at oblique axes

		Example 1	*Example 2*	*Example 3*
Sphere 1	S_1	1.00	0.00	0.00
Cylinder 1	F_1	1.00	2.00	3.00
Axis 1	A_1	0.00	60.00	0.00
Sphere 2	S_2	0.00	–3.00	0.00
Cylinder 2	F_2	–1.00	3.00	–3.00
Axis 2	A_2	120.00	120.00	30.00
Angle between cylinders	$a = A_2 - A_1$	120.00	60.00	30.00
	$\text{Tan } 2B = (F_2 \sin 2a)/(F_1 + F_2 \cos 2a)$	0.5774	5.1962	–1.7321
Angle B	$B = (\tan^{-1}(2B))/2$	15.00	39.55	–30.00
Induced sphere	$S = F_1 \sin 2B + F_2 \sin 2(B - a)$	–0.87	1.18	–1.50
Resultant sphere	$\text{Sphere} = S_1 + S_2 + S$	0.13	–1.82	–1.50
Resultant cylinder	$\text{Cylinder} = F_1 + F_2 - 2S$	1.73	2.65	3.00
*Resultant axis**	$\text{Axis} = A_1 + B$	15	100	150

*If resultant axis is negative, add 180 to give final answer
Note that the angle A_2 must be longer than the angle A_1 in standard notation.

If this expression is made equal to zero and differentiated, this gives the value of the relative axis of the cylinder as:

$$Tan\ 2B = \frac{F_2 \sin 2a}{F_1 + F_2 \cos 2a}$$

Assuming that we are finding the plus cylinder transposition, then the resultant sphere power can be found from:

$$S = F_1 \sin^2 B + F_2 \sin^2(a - B)$$

The resultant cylinder is:

$$C = F_1 + F_2 - 2S$$

Examples of the calculation method are shown in Table 3.5.

Summary

Lenses consisting of or incorporating cylinders are used to correct astigmatism. Astigmatism is a defect of an eye or lens system where a line image is produced from a point object due to differences in power in the principal meridians of the system. The theoretical aspects of cylindrical surfaces such as their radii and sag are discussed, as are the alternative standard notations for such lenses in both 'thick' and 'thin' forms.

Formulae

Formula	*Name*	*Equation number*
$r_\theta = r/\sin^2\theta$	Radius of cylindrical surface curvature at angle θ to axis	3.01
$r_\theta = r_v - [(r_v - r_h)/\cos\theta]$	Radius of curvature at a non-equatorial point on a toroidal surface	3.02

4

Prisms and prismatic effects

Prisms

In Chapter 1, a prism was defined as a lens causing deviation of light without changing its vergence. The deviation produced by a prism is given by:

$d = (n' - 1)a$ *Equation 1.10*

where a is the apical angle of the prism (Figure 1.15). More usually, the deviation produced by a prism is expressed in terms of its prismatic power, P, where:

$P = 100 \tan d$ *Equation 1.11*

The unit of prism power is the prism dioptre, given the symbol Δ. A prism with a power of 1 prism dioptre will deviate light by 1 centimetre measured at a distance of 1 metre from the prism (Figure 1.16). In other words, the SI unit of prismatic power is cm/m.

It can be seen from Equation 1.11 that the relationship between deviation and prismatic power is not a straightforward one. The deviation of light in degrees by a prism of 1 prism dioptre power is $d = \tan^{-1}(1/100) = 0.57°$. Further, the prism's apical angle is $a = 0.57/(n - 1) = 1°$ (to one significant figure) for crown glass. Also, the prismatic power of a prism that deviates light by 1° is $P = 100 \tan 1 = 1.74Δ$.

Identification of prisms

Prisms can be identified in several ways. First, a prism consists of two flat planes inclined at an angle to form an apex and a base. The base end of a prism is therefore thicker by inspection than the apex end. Secondly, a plano prism deviates light but does not change its vergence. Thus there will be no transverse ('with' or 'against') movement of an image when a lens is moved against an object.

Thirdly, a prism deviates the image of an object towards its apex. In Figure 4.1, a cross-line object is being viewed through a plano prism. In Figure 4.1a, the image is shown deviated towards the apex along the base–apex line. In Figure 4.1b, the prism has been rotated so that the base–apex line is vertical. At this point, the vertical object and image lines coincide, and the prism can be marked as shown, with a line along the base–apex direction. An arrow is used to indicate the apex of the prism, and a short transverse line the base. Figure 4.1c shows a cross-section of the prism, showing how the image is formed deviated towards the apex.

Prism orientation

Prisms can be orientated in front of the eye using standard axis notation (Figure 4.2). The angle indicates the position of the base, and as prisms are not symmetrical about their mid-point, the full 360° protractor must be used.

More commonly, prisms are only placed horizontally or vertically, and oblique angle prisms are produced by resolving the prism

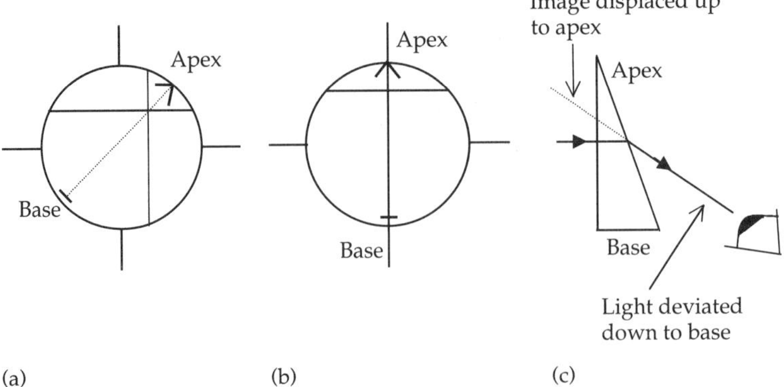

Figure 4.1. Deviation of an object by a prism. The prism always deviates the image towards its apex. Note the marking system for the prism: the arrowhead represents the apex and the short line the base.

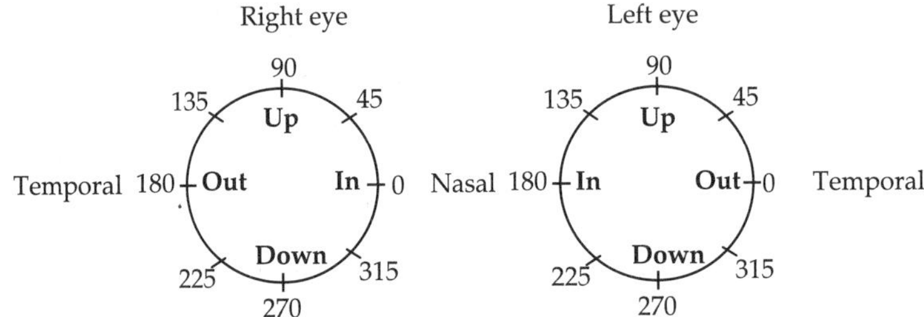

Figure 4.2. Standard notation for prism orientation, marked in both degrees and base direction. Note that 'In' and 'Out' do not have the same numerical value for base direction in right and left eyes.

into horizontal and vertical components. The prism is described as Base Up, Base Down, Base In or Base Out where 'In' refers to the nasal side of the eye (Figure 4.2).

Combining prisms

If prisms are combined with their base–apex lines parallel, and with their bases in the same direction, then their effects are considered to be additive, just as with thin lenses. For example, if 3Δ Base Up is combined with 2Δ Base Up, then the resultant effect will be 5Δ Base Up. On the other hand, if 3Δ Base Up is combined with 2Δ Base Down, then the resultant effect will be 1Δ Base Up.

If the base–apex lines of the two prisms to be combined are not parallel, then the single effective prism can be produced by resolving the two prisms. In Figure 4.3, two prisms are placed in front of a right eye. One is 3Δ Base Up (axis 90) and the other is 4Δ Base In (axis 360). From Pythagoras' theorem, the power of the single prism that would replace these two is: $\sqrt{(3^2 + 4^2)} = 5\Delta$. The base orientation is given by $\sin^{-1}(3/5) = 36.9°$. It is also possible to do the reverse calculation and find the two

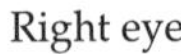

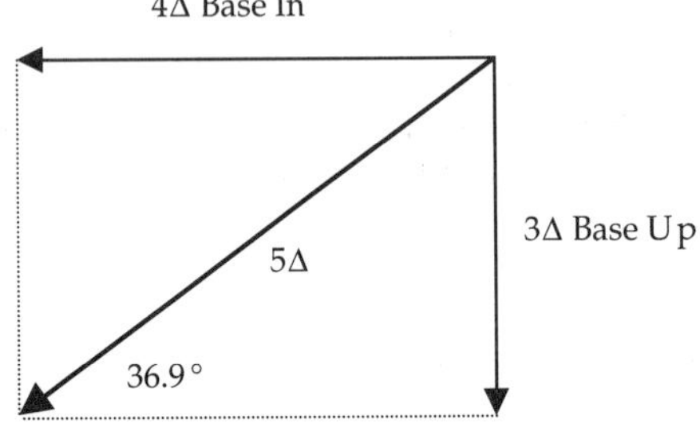

Figure 4.3. Resolution of two prisms. The arrows represent the apices of the prisms.

prisms aligned on major axes required to replace one oblique prism.

An instrument that uses the technique of resolving prisms to give a continuously variable prism is the Risley Rotary Prism. The instrument consists of two 15Δ plano-prisms held in a geared mounting. When the base–apex lines of the prisms are parallel and their bases are opposite, the resultant prismatic power is zero. When the base–apex lines are parallel and the bases are in the same direction, then the resultant power is the sum of the powers of the two prisms (30Δ). If the base–apex lines are not parallel, the prismatic power of each prism is given by $P \sin \theta$, where θ is the angle the prism has been rotated from the position of zero prismatic power. Risley rotary prisms are used in binocular vision for measuring and exercising fusional reserves. They may also be found in refractor heads and on focimeters.

Thickness differences in prisms

To produce a lens with both focal power and prismatic power, lenses are produced with one surface tilted relative to the other.

Figure 4.4 illustrates a section through the centre of a lens incorporating prism, along the base–apex line. The angle of the prism is a, the lens diameter d and the difference in edge

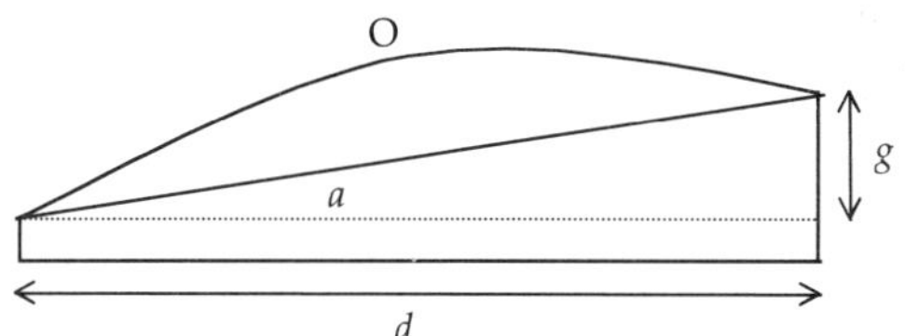

Figure 4.4. Workshop Prism Formula.

thickness along the base–apex line is g. The deviation produced by a small angle prism is:

$$\text{deviation} = (n' - 1)a \qquad \textit{Equation 1.10}$$

where both the induced deviation and the prism angle are in the same units, usually degrees. If we wished to express the angle of the prism in prism dioptres (Δ) then this could be expressed as $100\,g/d$, from the definition of a prism dioptre. Thus the deviation induced by a prism, P, in prism dioptres can be expressed as:

$$P = 100(n' - 1)g/d \qquad \textit{Equation 4.01}$$

where g and d are in the same units.

Equation 4.1 is known as the Workshop Prism Formula, and is used during the manufacture of prismatic lenses. By measuring the difference in edge thicknesses along the base–apex line, it enables the induced prism to be calculated before the lens is polished and optically transparent.

Note that in the workshop prism formula, the optical centre of the focal powered lens (O in the diagram) considered on its own is assumed to be at the centre of the lens, and the formula calculates the prism at the centre of the lens. The prismatic effect at any other point on the lens will have to take into account the decentration of the powered section.

Fresnel prisms

In anything greater than low prismatic powers, prisms have thick bases and become cosmetically unappealing. An alternative to adding working prisms onto spectacle lenses is to use Fresnel prisms. Fresnel prisms were originally designed for use in lighthouse beacons by Augustin Fresnel in the nineteenth century. Press-on Fresnel prisms for spectacle lenses became available in the 1970s (Adams *et al.*, 1971).

The Fresnel prism works on the principle that the prism apex deviates light just as much as any other part of the lens. A series of 'prism apices' on a thin base sheet are used to obtain a prismatic effect across the lens without creating additional lens thickness (Figure 4.5).

Fresnel prisms are moulded from PVC (polyvinylchloride) to form a flexible sheet of prism. The sheet is cut to the shape of the spectacle lens, and fixed with the smooth side attached to the rear surface of the lens with water. Since Fresnel prisms are easily attached and removed from lenses, they are used in preference to conventional prisms in the management of short-term or frequently changing binocular vision disorders.

Fresnel prisms compare favourably to conventional prisms in terms of cosmesis at high powers, since the thickness saving can be considerable. Fresnel prisms can be

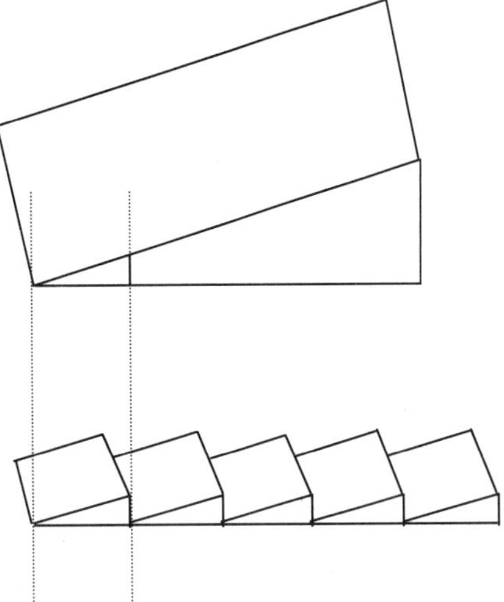

Figure 4.5. Principle of Fresnel prisms (after Adams *et al.*, 1971).

obtained in powers (up to 30Δ) that it would be difficult to incorporate using conventional prisms. However, the grooves between the strips of prism can be noticeable. Optically, Fresnel prisms show less overall image magnification than conventional prisms, and show similar effects to conventional prisms in terms of other distortions (Adams *et al.*, 1971).

Functionally, Fresnel prisms reduce visual acuity and contrast sensitivity, particularly for powers greater than 10Δ (Woo *et al.*, 1986). The reductions in function are mainly due to chromatic aberration, and are more pronounced for Fresnel prisms than for conventional prisms.

Prismatic effects of focal lenses

In Chapter 1 it was shown that even if a focal lens has no prism worked onto it, the lens has prismatic effects when viewed through points on the lens away from the optical centre. The relationship between the distance from the optical centre and the prismatic effect is given by Prentice's Rule:

$$P = cF \qquad \text{Equation 1.12}$$

If the optical centre of a lens is moved away from a given reference point, such as the patient's visual axis, the lens is said to be decentred. From Prentice's Rule, a decentred lens induces a prismatic effect.

Decentration of lenses

The decentration of a lens and its resultant prismatic effects can be calculated for spherical lenses and sphero-cylindrical lenses with the cylinders along the major axes (90° and 180°) using Prentice's Rule. The following points should be noted:

1. The direction of decentration is the direction of movement of the optical centre from the reference point (not the direction the reference point moves from the optical centre). For example, consider that the eyes move down to view an object on the floor. Since the optical centre now lies above the reference point, the direction of decentration is up.
2. Decentrations or prism bases that are downwards or outwards are given positive values in Prentice's Rule. Decentrations or prism bases that have an inwards or upwards direction are given negative values. A convenient phrase to remember these sign conventions by is: *Down and Out are positive, Up and In are negative.*
3. Positive power lenses give prism bases in the same direction as decentration. In Figure 4.6a, the positive lens is considered as two prisms mounted base to base. When the lens is moved down, the image moves up towards the prism apex, and Base Down prism is induced.
4. Negative power lenses give prism bases in the opposite direction to decentration. In Figure 4.6b, the negative lens is considered as two prisms mounted apex to apex. When the lens is moved down, the image also moves down towards the prism apex, and Base Up prism is induced.

Figure 4.6 also explains the movements seen during hand neutralization (Chapter 6). A positive lens induces an 'against' movement (lens moves down, image moves up), while a negative lens gives a 'with' movement.

Example:
What prism will be induced if a +3.00 DS lens is decentred 3 mm up in front of an eye?

$P = cF$

$P = (-0.3) \times (+3)$

$P = -0.9$

$P = 0.9\Delta$ Base Up

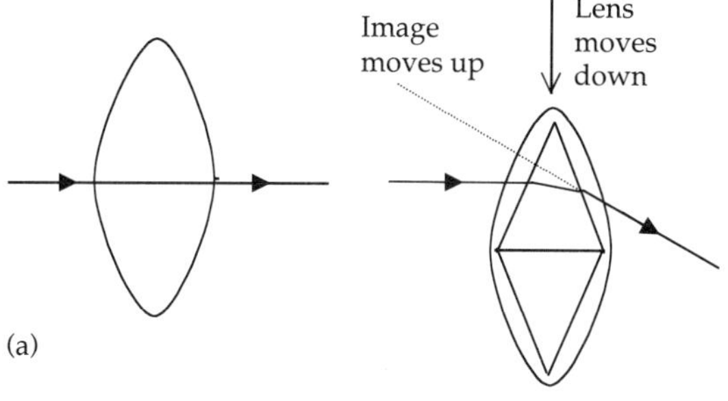

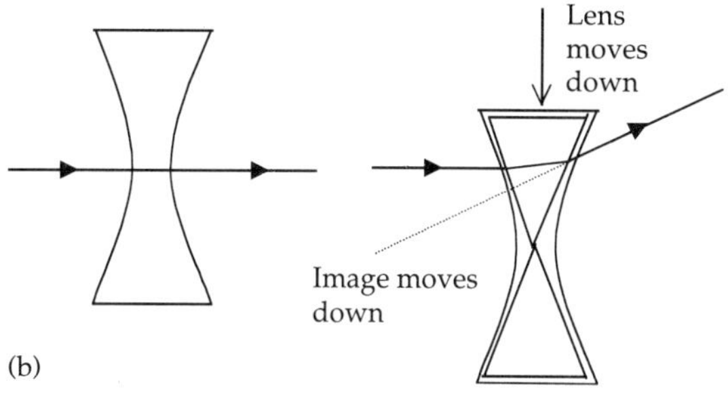

Figure 4.6. Transverse movements of lenses giving rise to decentration and prismatic effects: (a) positive lens; (b) negative lens.

Remember that decentration (c) should be specified in cm. A –3.00 DS lens would give 0.9Δ Base Down for decentration in the same direction.

For decentration of sphero-cylindrical prescriptions, the following apply:

1. A cylinder decentred along its axis will give no prismatic effect (Figure 4.7).
2. A cylinder decentred perpendicular to its axis will give a prismatic effect equivalent to a sphere of the same power (Figure 4.7).
3. The sphere and cylinder of a sphero-cylindrical prescription can be treated as two separate lenses.

Example:
What prism will be induced if a +3.00 DC × 180 lens is decentred 3 mm up in front of an eye?

The axis is horizontal, so vertical decentration (perpendicular to the axis) will give the maximum prismatic effect of 0.9Δ Base Up, as in the previous example. If the lens had been +3.00 DC × 90, vertical decentration along the cyl axis would have given no prismatic effect as there is no power in this meridian.

Example:
What is the induced prismatic effect when +3.00 DS/–4.00 DC × 90 is decentred 4 mm in and 2 mm up?

The calculation can be approached in two ways, either in the sphero-cyl form, or transposed to the cross-cyl form.

1. *Sphero-cyl method:*
   - Prism due to sphere:

     HΔ = cF = –0.4 × (+3) = –1.2 = 1.2Δ Base In
     VΔ = cF = –0.2 × (+3) = –0.6 = 0.6Δ Base Up

   - Prism due to cylinder:

     HΔ = cF = –0.4 × (–4) = +1.6 = 1.6Δ Base Out
     VΔ = cF = –0.2 × (0) = 0 = zero vertical prism

   - Overall prismatic effect:

     HΔ = –1.2 + 1.6 = +0.4 = **0.4Δ Base Out**
     VΔ = –0.6 + 0 = –0.6 = **0.6Δ Base Up**

2. *Cross-cyl method:*
   - Prescription in cross-cyl format is:

     +3.00 DC × 180/–1.00 DC × 90

   - Horizontally: $P = cF$ = (–0.4) × (–1) = +0.4 = **0.4Δ Base Out**
   - Vertically: $P = cF$ = (–0.2) × 3 = –0.6 = **0.6Δ Base Up**

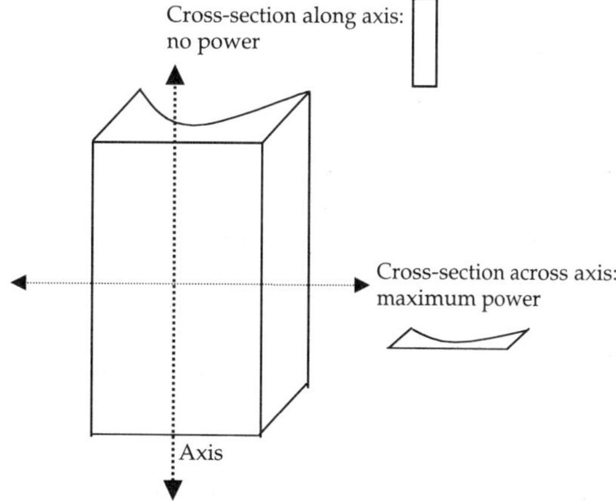

Figure 4.7. Decentration of a plano-cylinder. This is a negative cylinder, axis 90. If the lens is moved vertically along the axis there is no power and therefore no prismatic effect. Moving horizontally, or perpendicularly to the axis, there is maximum power and the prismatic effect is given by Prentice's Rule.

Decentration required to give specific prism

When prism is required to be incorporated into a prescription, this can be achieved either by grinding a lens incorporating a prism (see section on Workshop Prism Formula), or by decentration of a lens. Rearranging Prentice's Rule to the form: $c = P/F$ allows us to determine how much decentration would be required to provide a specific prismatic effect, if the prescription calls for both focal power and prism.

Example:
A prescription calls for +5.00 DS with 2Δ Base Out prism. What decentration is required to achieve this?

$c = P/F$

$c = (+2)/(+5) = +0.4$ cm = 4 mm Out

Note that although Prentice's Rule states decentration in cm, it is usual to quote answers in mm.

If the focal power is low or the prismatic power required is high, then too much decentration may be required to provide the prism in this way.

Example:
How much decentration would be required to give 4Δ Base Out on a +0.50 DS lens?

$c = P/F = (+4)/(+0.5) = +8$ cm = 80 mm Out

The maximum possible blank size of most modern lenses is about 80 mm, and so obviously 80 mm of decentration cannot be incorporated into a lens. In cases such as these, prism must be worked onto the lens using the Workshop Prism Formula. It should also be noted that prism should never be worked on aspheric lenses (Chapter 7) by decentration, as the patient should always look through the optical centre of these lenses. If prism is required in an aspheric lens, it must be produced by working the prism onto the lens.

Prism induced by decentration of a sphero-cylinder at any axis

So far we have considered only spherical prescriptions, and sphero-cylindrical prescriptions with cylinder axes on the major meridians (90° and 180°). What happens when a prescription with a cylinder at some other axis, such as 30°, is decentred up or out?

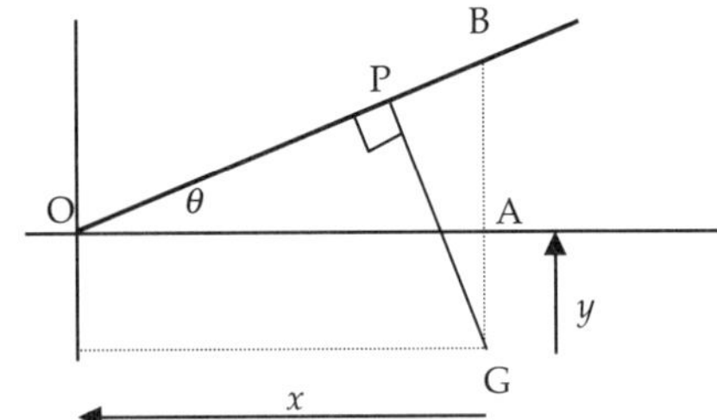

Figure 4.8. Graphical representation of a cylindrical lens at some axis θ to the horizontal, in order to calculate the decentration of a cylinder in horizontal and vertical terms.

To approach the problem, the sphere and cylinder are considered separately, and the decentration and power are defined for each element. Figure 4.8 shows graphically the cylindrical portion of the prescription, which is all that is considered initially. The diagram shows a cylinder of power C dioptres oriented at a general angle θ to the horizontal. The patient is looking through the lens at point G. The optical centre, O, has been decentred x cm horizontally and y cm vertically from this reference point. A perpendicular to the cylinder is shown as PG.

The first stage of the proof is to define PG in terms of the horizontal and vertical decentration (x and y).

Since angle PGA = θ

$$PG = BG \cos\theta = (BA + y)\cos\theta$$

Also, $\tan\theta = BA/x$

$$PG = (x\tan\theta + y)\cos\theta$$

From trigonometry, $\tan\theta = \sin\theta/\cos\theta$

$$PG = (x\sin\theta/\cos\theta + y)\cos\theta = (x\sin\theta + y\cos\theta)$$

PG is now resolved into horizontal and vertical components (Figure 4.9) to give the horizontal and vertical decentrations due to the cylindrical portion of the prescription.

$\sin\theta = \text{Horizontal } c/PG$

$\text{Horizontal } c = PG\sin\theta$

$\text{Horizontal } c = (x\sin\theta + y\cos\theta)\sin\theta$

$\cos\theta = \text{Vertical } c/PG$

$\text{Vertical } c = PG\cos\theta$

$\text{Vertical } c = (x\sin\theta + y\cos\theta)\cos\theta$

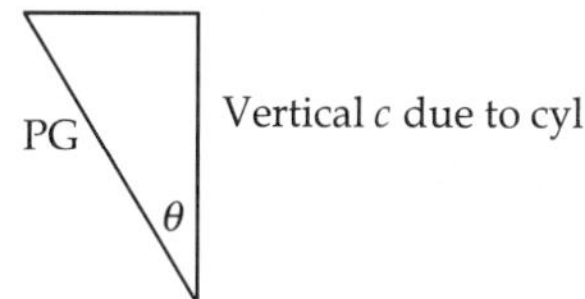

Figure 4.9. PG is resolved into horizontal and vertical components.

Finally, using Prentice's Rule, the horizontal and vertical prismatic effects are defined for the sphere and cylinder powers and added together to give overall horizontal and vertical prismatic effects. S represents the sphere power, in dioptres.

Horizontal Δ =
(cyl decentration × cyl power) + (sphere decentration × sphere power)

Horizontal Δ =
$(x \sin\theta + y \cos\theta) \sin\theta.\ C + x.S$ *Equation 4.02*

Vertical Δ =
(cyl decentration × cyl power) + (sphere decentration × sphere power)

Vertical Δ =
$(x \sin\theta + y \cos\theta) \cos\theta.\ C + y.S$ *Equation 4.03*

Strict sign conventions must be followed when attempting to determine prismatic effects using this type of calculation. The sign conventions are summarized as follows:

- For axis notation: L axis (θ) = standard notation; R axis (θ) = 180 – standard notation. The reason for θ being defined differently in the two eyes is that standard notation has zero on the nasal side of the right eye, but on the temporal side of the left eye (Figure 4.2).
- As previously, the sign assigned to values is given by: Down and Out are positive; Up and In are negative. These sign conventions hold for prism base direction and the direction the optical centre has moved away from the point of viewing (NOT the direction the viewing point has moved from the optical centre).

Example:
What is the prismatic effect in the following lens?

Left eye: –2.25 DS/–2.00 DC × 40 3 mm Out

1. First, identify the decentration of the OC in cm:

   $x = +0.3$ (Note the value is positive because the decentration is 'out')

   $y = 0$

2. Next, identify the sphere and cyl powers:

   S = –2.25

   C = –2

3. Finally, identify the axis:

   $\theta = 40$ (Note it is a left eye, so the axis is in standard notation.)

Having identified all the parameters, insert these into the relevant equations (Equations 4.02 and 4.03):

$H\Delta = (x \sin\theta + y \cos\theta) \sin\theta.\ C + x.S$

$H\Delta = [[(0.3 \times \sin 40) + (0)] \times (\sin 40 \times (-2))] + (0.3 \times (-2.25))$

$H\Delta = -0.92$

HΔ = 0.92Δ Base In

$V\Delta = (x \sin\theta + y \cos\theta) \cos\theta.\ C + y.S$

$V\Delta = [[(0.3 \times \sin 40) + (0)] \times (\cos 40 \times (-2))] + 0$

$V\Delta = -0.29$

VΔ = 0.29Δ Base Up

It is important to note that although there is no vertical decentration, vertical prism is induced. Both horizontal and vertical prismatic effects should always be calculated for oblique axis sphero-cylindrical prescriptions.

Decentration required to give prism for any sphero-cylinder

The decentration required to give a specific prismatic effect has been calculated so far from $c = P/F$, for spherical and sphero-cylindrical prescriptions with the cylinder on a major axis. It is also useful to be able to calculate the decentration required for a prismatic effect with any axis of cylinder.

Taking the previously derived equations:

$H\Delta = (x \sin\theta + y \cos\theta)$
$\sin\theta.\ C + x.S$ *Equation 4.02*

$V\Delta = (x \sin\theta + y \cos\theta)$
$\cos\theta.\ C + y.S$ *Equation 4.03*

Rearrange to make x and y the subject of the equations:

$$H\Delta = C.x.\sin^2\theta + C.y.\sin\theta.\cos\theta + x.S$$

$$V\Delta = C.x.\sin\theta.\cos\theta + C.y.\cos^2\theta + y.S$$

$$H\Delta = x(C.\sin^2\theta + S) + y(C.\sin\theta.\cos\theta)$$

$$V\Delta = x(C.\sin\theta.\cos\theta) + y(C.\cos^2\theta + S)$$

Then let:

$$A = S + C.\sin^2\theta \qquad \textit{Equation 4.04}$$

$$B = C.\sin\theta.\cos\theta \qquad \textit{Equation 4.05}$$

$$D = S + C.\cos^2\theta \qquad \textit{Equation 4.06}$$

Substituting Equations 4.04–4.06 into the previously derived expressions gives:

$$H\Delta = Ax + By$$

$$V\Delta = Bx + Dy$$

Solving these equations simultaneously gives:

$$y = \frac{H - Ax}{B} = \frac{V - Bx}{D}$$

$$DH - ADx = BV - B^2x$$

$$(AD - B^2)x = DH - BV$$

$$x = \frac{DH - BV}{AD - B^2}$$

$$AD - B^2 = [(S + C\cos^2\theta)(S + C\sin^2\theta)] - (C\sin\theta\cos\theta)^2$$

$$= S^2 + SC\sin^2\theta + SC\cos^2\theta + (C\sin\theta\cos\theta)^2 - (C\sin\theta\cos\theta)^2$$

Since $\sin^2\theta + \cos^2\theta = 1$

$$AD - B^2 = S(S + C)$$

$$x = \frac{DH - BV}{S(S + C)} \qquad \textit{Equation 4.07}$$

Also:

$$x = \frac{H - By}{A} = \frac{V - Dy}{B}$$

$$BH - B^2y = AV - ADy$$

$$(AD - B^2)y = AV - BH$$

$$y = \frac{AV - BH}{S(S + C)} \qquad \textit{Equation 4.08}$$

Note that if $(S(S + C))$ equates to zero, then there is no possible solution. There are some special cases where solutions are possible, such as when the cylinder axis is 90° or 180° and Prentice's Rule can be used, or when the decentration is along the cylinder axis.

Example:
A right lens has the prescription +0.25 DS/ +0.25 DC × 25. A prism of power 4Δ Base Down is required. What decentration would be required to achieve this?

1. First, identify the prismatic effect required:

   $H = 0$

   $V = +4$

2. Next, identify the sphere and cyl powers:

   $S = +0.25$

   $C = +0.25$

3. Finally, identify the axis:

   $\theta = 155$

Note it is a right eye, so the axis is (180 – standard notation).

Having identified all the parameters, insert these into the relevant equations:

$$A = S + C.\sin^2\theta$$

$$A = 0.295$$

$$B = C.\sin\theta.\cos\theta$$

$$B = -0.096$$

$$D = S + C.\cos^2\theta$$

$$D = 0.455$$

$$S(S + C) = 0.125$$

$x = (DH - BV)/S(S + C) = 3.07 = 30.7$ mm out

$y = (-BH + AV)/S(S + C) = +9.44 = 94.4$ mm down

Relative prismatic effects

When prisms are placed in front of one eye, the effects of combining prisms are simply additive. For example, 2Δ Base Up combined with 3Δ Base Down will give an overall effect of 1Δ Base Down.

When prisms are placed in front of both eyes, the effects depend on whether the base setting of the prisms is horizontal or vertical. The relative prismatic effect, or differential prism, can be defined as the single prism placed in front of one eye that will give the same effect as prisms placed before each of the two eyes.

- Horizontal: same bases additive; opposite bases subtractive
- Vertical: same bases subtractive; opposite bases additive.

For vertical prism therefore, the eye to which the prism is applied must be specified.

Example:
A prism of 2Δ Base Down is required for the left eye. An equivalent way of providing this prism is to give 2Δ Base Up right eye. Another more usual way of prescribing this prism would be to divide it equally between the eyes, giving 1Δ Base Up right eye and 1Δ Base Down left eye. If by error the prescription was made up as 1Δ Base Up right eye and 1Δ Base Up left eye, then the two vertical prisms would cancel, giving zero relative prismatic effect.

Example:
What is the relative prismatic effect for the following prescription:

RE: 2Δ Base In, 2Δ Base Up.

LE: 2Δ Base In, 2Δ Base Down.

Horizontally: 2 In + 2 In = 4Δ Base In

Vertically: 2 Up Right + 2 Down Left = 4Δ Base Up Right Eye OR 4Δ Base Down Left Eye.

Use of prisms

When a prism is placed monocularly in front of one eye, the eye rotates towards the prism apex, since the light is deflected towards the base and the image appears to have come from the apex. For example, if a Base Out prism is placed in front of an eye, the eye moves inwards; similarly, the eye moves outwards with a Base In prism in place.

If prism is placed binocularly in front of both eyes of a subject, the ocular movements depend on the relative prismatic effect. For example, with 2Δ Base Out in front of the right eye and 2Δ Base In in front of the left eye, the eyes move towards the apices of each prism, which is to the left in each case. Zero relative prism therefore gives rise to version movements of the eyes, where the angle between the visual axes of the two eyes does not change. However, if 2Δ Base Out is placed in front of both right and left eyes, the movement of both eyes is inwards, causing convergence of the eyes. Placing 2Δ Base In in front of each eye would cause divergence. For vertical prisms, the same base direction in front of each eye causes a version movement, while opposite prism bases in front of each eye give rise to vergence movements. In other words, relative prism gives rise to vergence movements of the eyes, where the angle between the visual axes of the eyes changes in order to maintain single binocular vision.

Prisms are used in spectacles in order to alleviate symptoms associated with disorders of binocular vision by deviating light to fall on the foveae of both eyes. It should be noted that prisms do not solve the underlying problem, but, by allowing images to fall on (or nearer to) the two foveae, prisms reduce symptoms and can allow comfortable single binocular vision. When prescribed in spectacles, prism can cause reduction in visual acuity and contrast sensitivity due to the effects of chromatic aberration (Woo *et al.*, 1986).

Practical considerations with prisms and prismatic effects

Prisms can also cause a number of unwanted effects. Unwanted prismatic effects in spectacles generally occur as a result of inappropriate positioning of the optical centres of the lenses, giving rise to decentration, prismatic effect and relative prismatic effects between the two eyes. Consider the fusional reserves, or vergence amplitudes, listed in Table 4.1. These values represent the amount of prism that can typically be placed before the two eyes before single binocular vision is lost and double vision occurs. It can be seen that vertical fusional reserves are very small, and so even small amounts of unprescribed relative vertical prism can cause symptoms of

Table 4.1 Normal fusional reserves (prism dioptres) (Evans, 1997)

	Convergence	*Divergence*	*Vertical*
Distance	15–23	5–9	2–4
Near	18–24	18–24	2–4

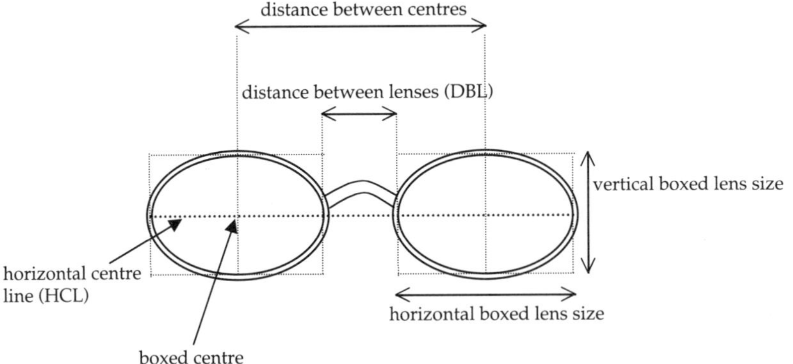

Figure 4.10. The boxed lens system of spectacle measurement.

asthenopia (eye strain), blurring or double vision. Relative vertical prismatic effects in spectacles should preferably be below 1Δ and certainly below 2Δ. Further, unwanted relative horizontal or vertical prism in binocular vision can reduce visual function as measured using contrast sensitivity (Tunnacliffe and Williams, 1985, 1986). Only 1Δ Base Down under photopic conditions, or 1/2Δ Base Down under mesopic conditions, can significantly reduce contrast sensitivity at all spatial frequencies.

In order to understand the situations where unwanted prismatic effects commonly arise, it is necessary to digress slightly and define the system of measurements used when prescribing spectacles. In the UK, the boxed lens system is used to measure spectacle parameters (BS3521 Part 2, 1991; BS EN ISO 8624: 1997. The basic frame measurements are shown in Figure 4.10, and facial measurements are shown in Figure 4.11. If the distance between centres of a frame and the interpupillary distance (PD) of a patient are the same value, then the patient's eyes look through the boxed centres of the lenses. Assuming that the optical centres of the lenses are coincident with the boxed centres, there are no prismatic effects for distance viewing. If the PD and the distance between centres have different values, then prismatic effects may be a problem, as shown in the following example.

Example:

In Figure 4.12, a patient has chosen a frame that has a horizontal boxed lens size of 60 mm and a distance between lenses of 20 mm. The patient's PD is 70 mm, and his prescription is –5.00 DS right and left.

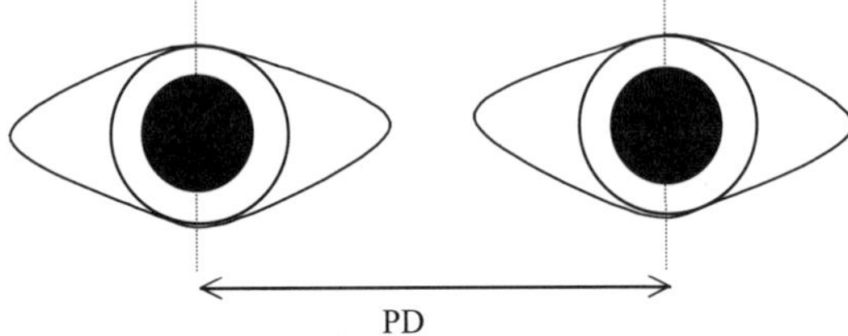

Figure 4.11. Interpupillary distance measurement for distance fixation (PD).

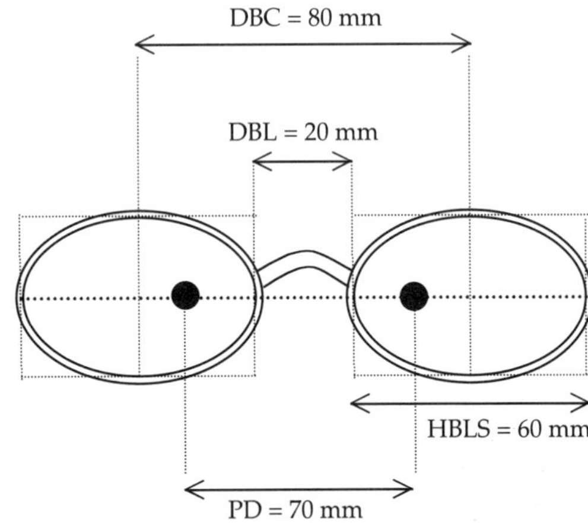

Figure 4.12. Unwanted prismatic effects induced in a spectacle frame where the distance between centres does not equal the PD of the patient. The optical centres of the lenses must be decentred away from the boxed centres of the frame to compensate.

The distance between centres of the lenses is 60 + 20 = 80 mm. However, the patient's PD is only 70 mm. Therefore, if the lenses are not decentred from the boxed centres, the patient will not look through the optical centres of the lenses. The optical centres are decentred 5 mm out from each of the patient's eyes, assuming the eyes are symmetrical and have equal monocular PDs.

From Prentice's Rule, $P = cF = (+0.5) \times (-5) = 2.5\Delta$ Base In per eye. A relative prismatic effect of 5Δ Base In is induced.

In order to centre the lenses correctly, the optical centres must be moved in by 5 mm per eye; i.e.

- Decentration per eye (Binocular measurements) = (PD – distance between centres)/2
- Decentration per eye (Monocular measurements) = monocular PD – (distance between centres/2)

Once the lenses are correctly centred for distance, the prismatic problems are not necessarily solved. Consider, for example, the single vision prescription of –5.00 DS right and left, prescribed for a young myope. The lenses are centred correctly for distance viewing, but the patient wears the spectacles full time. What likely prismatic effects at near will he experience?

When the eyes move to look at a near object, they generally converge and move down. Therefore, the eyes will not look through the optical centres in either the horizontal or vertical meridians. In a typical example the patient's eyes converge by 4 mm and he looks through a point on the lens 10 mm below the optical centre. The monocular prismatic effects are therefore:

- Horizontally: $P = cF = (-0.2) \times (-5) = 1\Delta$ Base Out R & L
- Vertically: $P = cF = (1) \times (-5) = 5\Delta$ Base Up R & L.

Binocularly, the relative prismatic effect is 2Δ Base Out. There is no vertical prismatic effect since the Base Up prisms in each eye cancel each other out.

In the examples above it was the decentration, *c*, which caused the problems with unwanted prismatic effect. Prismatic effects can also be due primarily to the power of the lenses, *F*. Consider an anisometropic patient with a single vision prescription of –5.00 DS in the right eye and plano in the left eye. The lenses are correctly centred for distance. What prismatic effects will the patient experience at near? If we consider that the eyes converge by 4 mm and look through a point 10 mm below the optical centre, as in the previous example, then the prismatic effects are:

- Horizontally:
  Right eye: $P = cF = (-0.2) \times (-5) = 1\Delta$ Base Out
  Left eye: $P = (-0.2) \times (0) = 0$
- Vertically:
  Right eye: $P = cF = (1) \times (-5) = 5\Delta$ Base Up
  Left eye: $P = 1 \times 0 = 0$

Binocularly, the relative prismatic effect is 1Δ Base Out, and 5Δ Base Up Right Eye. Recalling the extent of the fusional reserves (Table 4.1), it can be seen that the 5Δ vertical prismatic effect exceeds the 2Δ of vertical prism that the visual system can tolerate. The patient may experience asthenopia with these spectacles at near and need some form of prism compensation. Differential vertical prismatic effects are a particular problem with bifocals (see Chapter 8).

Binocular horizontal movements of the eyes (version movements) to look out of the edge of a spectacle lens do not generally cause problematic prismatic effects. So long as the lens power in each eye is the same, the prismatic effects in right and left eyes will cancel one another out (e.g. 2Δ Base In R and 2Δ Base Out L = zero relative prism). If the prescription is anisometropic, then some horizontal relative prismatic effect will be caused. Since horizontal fusional reserves are much larger than vertical reserves, any prismatic effect induced is unlikely to cause problems unless the prism exacerbates an existing binocular vision problem.

Minimum size uncut

When glazing a lens into a frame, it is obviously vital that the uncut lens is large enough to occupy the whole of the lens shape. The smallest uncut size necessary depends on the size and shape of the finished lens. If the finished lens is also to be decentred, then this will also affect the smallest uncut, or blank, size from which the finished lens can be cut.

Example:
A prescription of +6.00 DS 3Δ Base In is required. The patient has chosen a frame that

Table 4.2 Centration tolerance for glazed lenses incorporating less than 2Δ of prescribed prism, according to BS2738–1, 1998

Meridional lens powers (D)	*Horizontal tolerance*	*Vertical tolerance*
Both lenses: power < 2.00	0.25Δ and 2.0 mm displacement	0.25Δ and 1.0 mm total displacement
Both lenses: power ≥ 2.00	2.0 mm total displacement	1.0 mm total displacement
One lens < 2.00, and one lens ≥ 2.00	0.12Δ and 2.0 mm displacement	0.12Δ and 1.0 mm total displacement

requires the finished lens to be circular with a diameter of 48 mm. The prescription must be correct at the centre of this lens. What diameter circular uncut lens would be required if the prism were to be produced by decentration?

First, calculate the decentration required to give the desired prism:

$c = P/F$

$c = -3/+6 = -0.5 = 5$ mm In

To calculate the size of uncut required, consider Figure 4.13. In the diagram, the reference point G is the point the patient will look through and is at the centre of the finished lens, which has a radius of 24 mm. The optical centre O is decentred 5 mm in from G, as calculated above. Thus the optical centre is the centre of a circle of radius 29 mm. Therefore the minimum uncut diameter required is 58 mm. In practice, another 2 mm or so will be allowed for edging the lens.

In summary, the formula for calculating the minimum size uncut is as follows:

Minimum size uncut (MSU) =
maximum visible lens aperture +
(2 × decentration) + wastage *Equation 4.09*

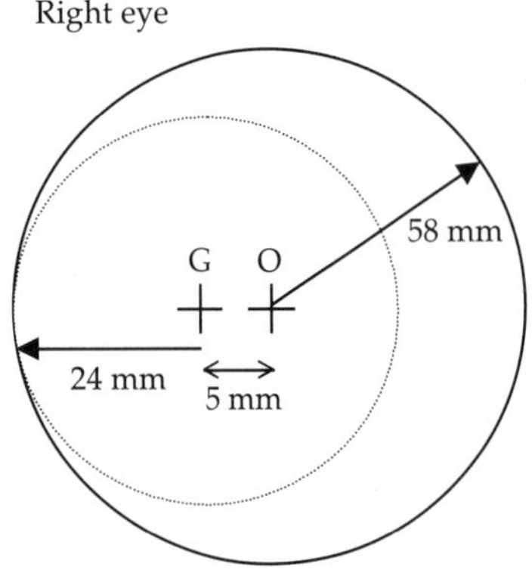

Figure 4.13. Calculation of minimum blank size or minimum uncut size.

Calculation of blank size in this way is often required for exaggerated lens shapes, and in cases where the distance between centres of the frame and the PD of the patient differ.

Tolerances on prism

The allowed tolerances on prismatic power depend on whether the lens is glazed or unglazed; whether the lens is single vision, multifocal or progressive; whether prismatic effect at the centration point or prescribed prism is being measured; and whether the prism is horizontal or vertical.

The tolerances allowed on optical centration and prescribed prism in glazed lenses are defined in BS 2738 Part 1 (1998). The tolerances on the position of the optical centre (or, for multifocal lenses, the distance optical centre) when less than 2Δ of prism is prescribed in each lens are shown in Table 4.2. Additional tolerances where prescribed prism is more than 2Δ are shown in Table 4.3.

Table 4.3 Additional tolerance for glazed lenses incorporating more than 2Δ of prescribed prism, according to BS2738–1, 1998

Relative prismatic power (Δ)	*Additional tolerance (Δ)*
> 2.00 and ≤ 10.00	± 0.37
>10.00	± 0.50

Summary

Prisms are lenses that deviate light towards their apices without changing vergence. Prisms are used to alleviate binocular vision problems. Lenses have prismatic effects when viewed through any other point on the lens than the optical centre. Such effects may be wanted or unwanted. Care must be taken when centring lenses that unwanted prismatic effects are not induced, particularly vertical differential prism, as they may disrupt binocular vision. Methods have been detailed by which to calculate prismatic effects of decentration, or decentration required to give specific prismatic effects.

Equations

Formula	*Name*	*Equation number*
$d = (n' - 1)a$	Deviation of light by prism	1.10
$P = 100\tan d$		1.11
$P = cF$	Prentice's Rule	1.12
$P = 100(n' - 1)g/d$	Workshop Prism Formula	4.01
Horizontal $\Delta = (x \sin\theta + y\cos\theta)\sin\theta.C + x.S$	Horizontal prism from decentration	4.02
Vertical $\Delta = (x \sin\theta + y\cos\theta)\cos\theta.C + y.S$	Vertical prism from decentration	4.03
$A = S + C.\sin^2\theta$		4.04
$B = C.\sin\theta.\cos\theta$		4.05
$D = S + C.\cos^2\theta$		4.06
$x = \dfrac{DH - BV}{S(S + C)}$	Decentration required for specific prism	4.07
$y = \dfrac{AV - BH}{S(S + C)}$	Decentration required for specific prism	4.08
MSU = maximum lens diameter required + (2 × decentration) + wastage	Minimum size uncut	4.09

Examples

Questions

1. A prism made of 1.7 index glass deviates light by 0.7°. What is the apical angle of the prism?
2. What is the power of the prism in question 1?
3. Light is shone through a prism of power 2Δ onto a screen positioned 1 m from the prism. By how much is the light deviated at the screen?
4. An object is viewed through the geometric centre of a right spectacle lens. The image is displaced to the left. What is the base setting of the prism in this lens?
5. A spectacle lens is measured on a focimeter. The prismatic power in the left lens is measured as 3.6Δ with a base setting of 41.8°. What was the original prism prescribed?
6. Prism is worked onto a lens of diameter 50 mm and refractive index 1.5. The edge thickness at the top of the lens is 5 mm; at the bottom of the lens the edge thickness is 2 mm. What prism was worked onto the lens?
7. A lens is required to be made to the prescription: +0.50 DS 4Δ Base Down. Obviously this prism cannot be incorporated into the lens by decentration, and the prism is to be worked onto the lens. What is the difference in edge thickness across this lens if the lens is to be made of 1.5 index glass with a diameter of 50 mm? What is the total prismatic effect if an object is viewed through a point on the lens 10 mm below the nominal position of the optical centre for the focal lens?
8. The optical centre of a +10.00 DS lens is decentred 10 mm out and 5 mm up. What horizontal and vertical prism is induced?
9. What is the prismatic effect at a point 5 mm inwards and 3 mm below the optical centre of a +3.00 DS lens?
10. A left lens of power –6.00 DC × 180 is decentred 5 mm in and 10 mm down. What is the prismatic effect?
11. A lens of power +6.00 DC × 90 is required to have prism of 3Δ Base In and 5Δ Base Down in front of the left eye. What decentration is required? Why can this prism not be achieved entirely by decentration, and what could be done instead?
12. A lens of power +6.00 DS/–4.00 DC × 180 is prescribed for the left eye. The observer's visual axis passes through the optical centre of the lens for distance viewing. What is the prismatic effect when reading through a point on the lens 10 mm below and 5 mm in from the optical centre?
13. A right lens of the form –3.00 DC × 90/ –2.00 DC × 180 requires prism of 2Δ Base

In and 1Δ Base Down. What decentration is required?

14. Calculate the prismatic effects of the following lens when decentred as indicated:
Left –2.25/–2.00 × 40, 3 mm out
15. Calculate the prismatic effects of the following lens when decentred as indicated:
Right –10.25/+0.75 × 160, 4 mm in, 2 mm down
16. What are the prismatic effects of the following lens when viewed through a point 10 mm inwards and 5 mm below the optical centre?
Right –2.00/–3.50 × 135
17. What are the prismatic effects of the following lens when viewed through a point 10 mm inwards and 5 mm below the optical centre?
Left –4.50/–2.00 × 130
18. What is the relative prismatic effect in a pair of spectacles made using the lenses in questions 10 and 11?
19. Calculate the decentrations required to give the indicated prism: Right +3.00/–4.25 × 160, 3Δ Base Out
20. Calculate the decentrations required to give the indicated prism: Left +10.25/–0.25 × 45, 2Δ Base Out, 1Δ Base Down
21. Calculate the decentrations required to give the indicated prism: Right –14.25/+6.00 × 175, 6Δ Base In, 4Δ Base Up
22. A frame with a maximum visible aperture of 63 mm, horizontal boxed lens size of 60 mm and distance between lenses of 20 mm is to be dispensed to a patient with a PD of 70 mm. What decentration is required to place the optical centres of the lenses in front of the patient's eyes? What relative prismatic effect would be induced if the lenses were not decentred and the prescription is –5.00 DS R & L? What is the minimum blank size required to give exact centres?
23. If a +6.00 D lens (index 1.50) has been decentred 4 mm in, and the horizontal boxed lens size of the finished lens is 56 mm, what is the difference in edge thickness along the horizontal meridian?
24. A patient returns to the practice with his new spectacles (Rx –4.00 DS right and left) complaining of eyestrain. His PD is 56 mm. The OCs of the new spectacles are placed 70 mm apart. How much prism has the patient been wearing?
25. A frame has the following boxed dimensions: horizontal 54 mm, vertical 48 mm, maximum aperture 59 mm, DBL 16 mm. If the patient's PD is 64 mm, what is the minimum blank size required if no allowance is made for cutting and edging?

Answers

1. 1°
2. 1.22Δ
3. 2 cm
4. Base Out
5. 2Δ Base Up, 3Δ Base Out
6. 3Δ Base Up
7. 4 mm; 4.5Δ Base Down
8. 10Δ Base Out; 5Δ Base Up
9. 1.5Δ Base Out; 0.9Δ Base Up
10. 6Δ Base Up
11. 0.5 cm in
12. 3Δ Base Out; 2Δ Base Up
13. 0.67 cm out; 0.5 cm up
14. 0.92Δ Base In; 0.29Δ Base Up
15. 4.11Δ Base Out; 2.01Δ Base Up
16. 2.88Δ Base In; 0.13Δ Base Down
17. 6.17Δ Base In; 3.65Δ Base Down
18. 9.05Δ Base In; 3.52Δ Base Down Left eye
19. 0.60 cm out; 1.09 cm up
20. 0.20 cm out; 0.10 cm down
21. 0.44 cm out; 0.51 cm down
22. 5 mm in per lens; 5Δ Base In; 75 mm blank
23. 2.69 mm
24. 5.6Δ Base In
25. 65 mm

5

Spectacle lens materials and lens manufacture

A spectacle lens material must satisfy a number of conflicting requirements. Besides being transparent to visible wavelengths, and constant in properties (homogeneous), the material must not split light up into the constituent colours to any great extent, giving rise to chromatic aberration. A spectacle lens must also have a range of desirable mechanical properties:

1. *Hardness*. The material needs to be robust to withstand the rough handling of daily use and hence requires a hard surface. Soft materials can have a hard coating applied to improve this property, but if a very hard coating is applied to a soft substrate there is always the risk of the coating cracking. Related to this is the ability of the material to be worked in the laboratory. Very hard material will take longer to surface or edge, and *vice versa*.
2. *Ease of tinting*. Whereas at one time it was common to use glass dyed in the mass for tinted lenses, currently the vast majority of lenses are manufactured in 'white' form and subsequently tinted by surface coating.
3. *Resistance to chemical attack*. Not only should a lens material be impervious to normal domestic solvents, it should also be resistant to atmospheric chemical attack, as well as to skin secretions. Some materials in the past have been prone to attack by common chemical agents, for example fruit juice and tobacco smoke.
4. *No adverse reactions*. Lens material must not cause adverse reactions in the wearer.

Spectacle lens materials can be readily divided into two categories; glass and plastics. (Note the description *plastics* to describe a material, the more common *plastic* being recommended for use as an adjective to describe the property of any material.)

General properties of lens materials

Refractive index

The refractive index of a lens material is an indication of how much it bends light in the yellow-green region of the spectrum (sometimes called the mean refractive index), and is defined as the velocity of light *in vacuo* divided by the velocity of light in the material. In practice, the refractive index is measured in air, and for spectacle lenses the difference in refractive index is not significant (Chapter 1).

For lenses of high power it is obviously desirable for a material to bend light as much as possible, so that very steep curves, giving thick and heavy lenses, are avoided. However, there are problems with high refractive index materials, as we shall see later.

In the UK the mean refractive index (n_d) has traditionally been measured at a specified wavelength of 587.56 nm, which corresponds to the helium 'd' line. Unfortunately there is not yet universal agreement as to the wavelength for refractive index measurement, the use of 546.07 nm, corresponding to the mercury 'e' line (labelled as index n_e) being common in continental Europe. An international standard (BS EN ISO 7944: 1998) recognizes both wavelengths, but it is hoped that a revised version of this standard will settle on one wavelength. For commercial reasons this is likely to be that of the mercury *e* line. To put the matter in perspective, the values for three lens materials are shown in Table 5.1.

Table 5.1 Refractive indices of three lens materials

Material	Refractive indices	
	n_d	n_e
Ophthalmic crown	1.523	1.525
CR39	1.498	1.500
Corning D0035	1.700	1.704

The problem that this can cause is that a lens manufacturer may calculate the surfacing curves for a lens base on one refractive index, while a user may measure the same lens on a focimeter calibrated for another.

For example, if a plano-concave spectacle lens is manufactured with a BVP of –10.00 DS, using a crown glass material ($n_d = 1.523$), then this will have a radius of curvature for the concave surface of 52.3 mm. If this same lens is checked on a focimeter calibrated for the mercury line (n_e), then the power will read –10.04 DS. Thus for high power lenses it can be important to know the wavelength used for calculating the lens power.

Refractive index is measured by material manufacturers using specialized equipment, for example the Abbe refractometer (Freeman, 1990) in order to obtain a high precision of measurement for quality control. BS 3062: 1985 (an obsolete, but still available, standard mainly for glass materials) specifies a tolerance in refractive index of ±0.001 for values up to 1.59, +0.001–0.0015 for the range over 1.59 to 1.69, and ±0.0015 for values over 1.69.

Constringence

This value is sometimes known as the Abbe number, and relates the refractive index of the material in the yellow-green region of the visible spectrum to the values at the blue and red ends. An ideal material would have a constant refractive index right across the visible spectrum. Unfortunately, all practical materials have a refractive index that varies with the wavelength.

In BS EN ISO 7944: 1998, constringence is determined by measuring the following values:

Source	Line	Symbol	Wavelength (nm)
Hydrogen (red)	C	n_C	656.27
Helium	d	n_d	587.56
Hydrogen (blue)	F	n_F	486.13

The constringence value (V_d) is then defined as:

$$V_d = \frac{n_d - 1}{n_F - n_C}$$

In technical optics it is more common to use the term *dispersive power*, which is the reciprocal of constringence.

As will be shown later, the constringence of a material tends to decrease as the refractive index increases. The practical significance of a low constringence is that it indicates a wide range of values for refractive index across the visible spectrum, giving rise to chromatic dispersion in a prism (Figure 5.1). In a lens, there are two types of chromatic aberration recognized, axial and transverse, depending on whether the incident light is parallel to the optical axis or oblique.

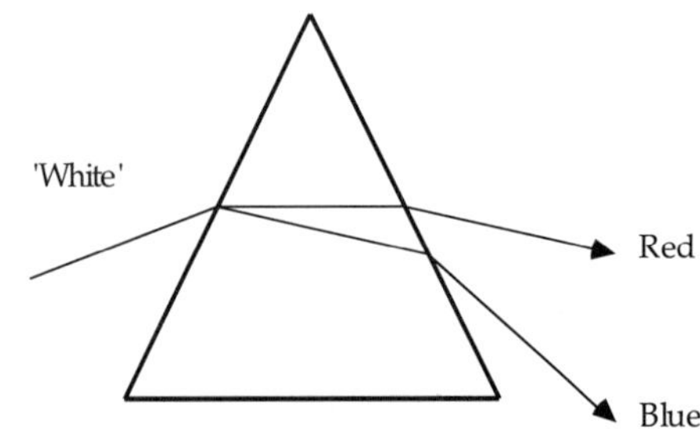

Figure 5.1. Dispersion by a plane prism.

To a first approximation, axial chromatic aberration (ACA) can be expressed as (in dioptres):

$$ACA = \frac{F}{V}$$

Thus for a +10.00 DS lens with a V of 60 the ACA would be 1/6 D, and, for a V of 30, 1/3 D. It might be asked how accurate this approximation is. Thus if we take a lens made of ophthalmic crown glass having a value of n_d of 1.523 and a BVP of +10.00 DS as above, and carry out an accurate ray trace, then typical values for the blue and red refractive indices would be $n_F = 1.5256$ and $n_C = 1.5169$. These values give a lens power of +10.054 D for blue light and +9.886 D for red, an overall axial chromatic aberration of 0.177 D. The approximate formula gives a value of 0.167 D.

Axial chromatic aberration does not constitute much of a problem in spectacle lenses because it is generally masked by considerable ACA exhibited by the human eye, which is of the order of 0.75 D.

In a similar fashion, transverse chromatic aberration can be calculated from the expression:

$$TCA = \frac{F}{V} y \quad (\Delta)$$

where 'y' is the distance from the optical centre in cm. The value calculated is in prism dioptres, and the expression is analagous to Prentices' rule for finding the prismatic effect of decentration. Thus in the case of a +5.00 DS lens, $V = 60$, at point 20 mm from the optical centre, the TCA would be 0.167Δ, and at 30 mm from the optical centre, 0.25Δ. Again, if the value of V was halved to 30, then the resulting TCA would be doubled.

To give an idea of the accuracy of this approximation, an accurate ray trace was again carried out. CR39 plastics material has a V of 59.3, thus at 20 mm from the OC, the TCA for a +5.00 DS lens by the expression given above would be 0.167Δ. Taking a +5.00 DS lens of 5.0 mm thickness, and rotating an eye 35° at 27 mm behind the rear surface, this would give an intersection distance with the front surface of 19.94 mm. The difference in deviation for the blue and red indices of 1.5040 and 1.4956 respectively gives a deviation of 0.181Δ.

Clinically the effects of TCA are to increase the blurring of images viewed through the periphery of a lens, and in severe cases to cause coloured fringing at high contrast boundaries in the visual field – window frames being a typical example. It is very difficult to predict the subjective acceptability of materials showing high dispersion. Many wearers accept the chromatic effects as a trade-off for having a thinner lens in a higher refractive index material.

BS 3062: 1985 sets tolerances on constringence of ±0.5 for values up to 45, and ±1.0 for values over 45.

Lens weight

There is a simple choice to be made with lens weight – for light lenses use plastics materials. In general plastics lenses are approximately half the weight of their glass counterparts. However, this simple approach conceals a more complex situation. The densities of both glass and plastics materials vary quite widely, as shown in Table 5.2.

Table 5.2 Lens materials

Name	n	V	*Density (g cm^{-3})*
Glass			
Crown	1.523	58	2.54
SW60	1.600	41	2.58
SF64	1.701	30	2.99
BaSF64	1.701	39	3.20
OF8035	1.800	35	3.56
Corning 1.9	1.885	31	3.99
Plastics			
Acrylic (PMMA)	1.491	58	1.19*
CR39	1.498	58	1.32
Polycarbonate	1.586	30	1.20*
HL–II	1.560	40	1.27
Super 16	1.600	34	1.37
Teslalid	1.710	36	1.40

* Thermoplastic material

It is not enough to compare lens weight and thickness simply on the basis of BVP. Other factors need to be taken into consideration, such as finished lens thickness and lens form. Figure 5.2 shows a comparison of lens weights for three common lens materials. These values were calculated for circular uncut lenses, all made in plano-convex form with a fixed 1.0 mm edge thickness. The three lens materials used were:

Material	n_d	V_d	*Density (g cm^{-3})*
White ophthalmic crown glass	1.523	58	2.54
High index glass	1.700	30	2.99
CR39 plastic	1.498	59	1.32

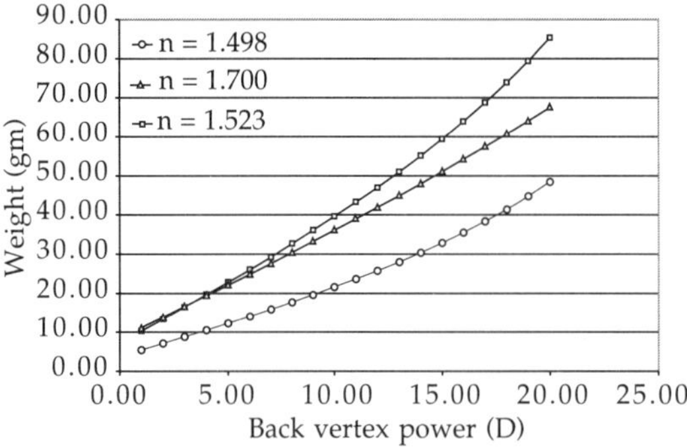

Figure 5.2. Calculated thicknesses for a series of lenses made in materials CR39 (n = 1.498, density 1.32 gm cm^{-3} crown glass (n = 1.523, density 2.54 gm cm^{-3}, and high index glass (n = 1.700, density 2.99 gm cm^{-3}. All lenses: 60 mm diameter, plano rear surface, 1.0 mm edge thickness (from Charman, 1991, with permission).

It will be apparent from Figure 5.2 that although the high-index glass is denser than crown, which is reflected in heavier lenses at low powers, at higher powers it actually gives lighter lenses. This is because the higher refractive index requires a smaller volume of lens material as a result of the flatter front surface curve on the lens. It should be pointed out, though, that except at very high powers this weight saving is relatively small, and patients should not be promised significantly lighter lenses when using high refractive index glass.

The graphs for lens thickness (Figure 5.3) are more straightforward, lens thickness on the graphs being in order of refractive index for the conditions given here, where plus lenses are compared finished to a common edge thickness of 1.0 mm.

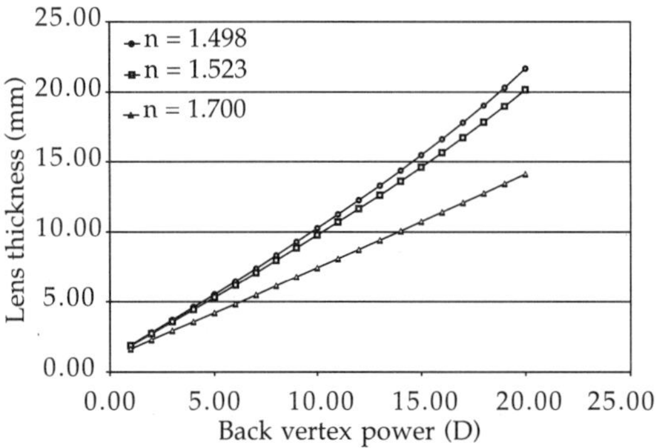

Figure 5.3. Calculated weights for lenses with the same characteristics as in Figure 5.2 (from Charman, 1991, with permission).

A comparison of minus power lenses is more difficult to make, as these are not made to a standard centre thickness. CR39 lenses in negative powers are generally produced to a minimum thickness of 2.0 mm, in order to retain mechanical stability. By comparison, glass lenses are surfaced down to 1.0 mm or so at high minus powers. What is advisable as a centre thickness in minus lenses is a complex question, as thicker lenses will be less prone to accidental breakage, whereas thinner lenses will look better and weigh less. It will be noticed that some modern high-index plastic materials are more rigid than CR39 and can be made to a centre thickness in the order of 1.0 mm in higher powers.

Flat form lenses will always be thinner and lighter than meniscus forms, as shown in Figure 5.4. As the meniscus form becomes steeper, this gives rise to steadily thicker and heavier lenses.

As lenses increase in diameter, they will naturally become thicker and heavier for a

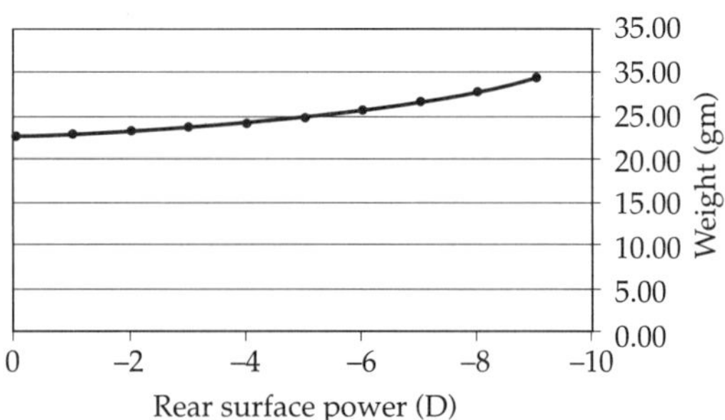

(a)

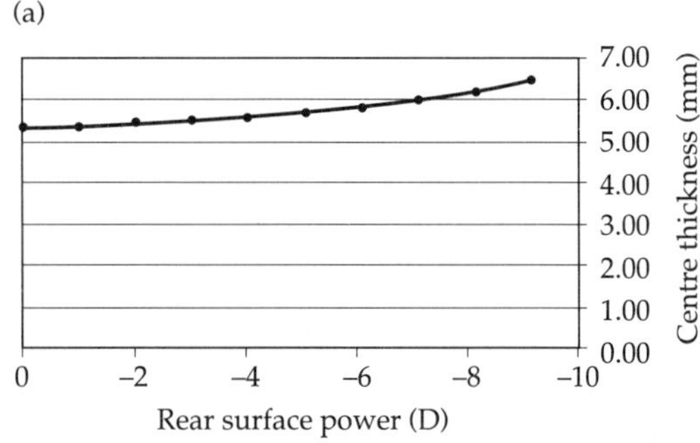

(b)

Figure 5.4. Effects of varying lens form on (a) the weight and (b) the thickness of 60-mm + 5.00 DS lenses manufactured in crown glass material (density 2.54 gm cm^{-3}, n = 1.523) with edge thickness of 1.0 mm.

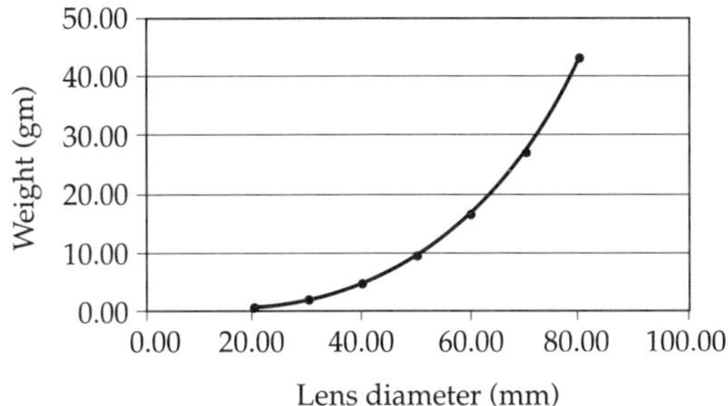

(a)

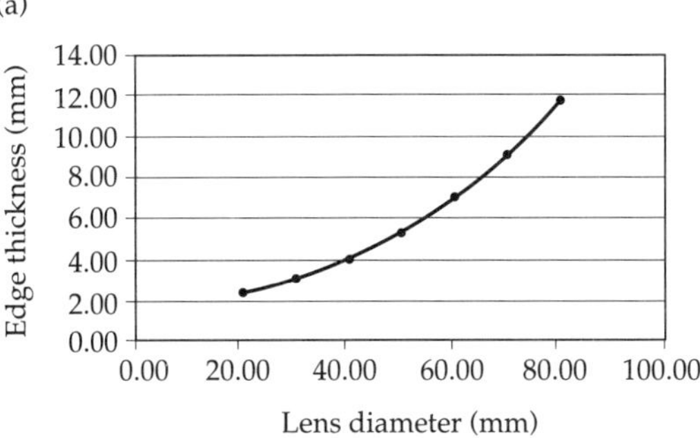

(b)

Figure 5.5. Effect of lens diameter on (a) weight and (b) edge thickness of a –5.00 DS lens made in CR39 material (density 1.32 gm cm^{-3}, n = 1.498), centre thickness 2.0 mm, front surface power +3.00 D.

given power (Figure 5.5). However, the *rate* of increase can be very considerable, particularly in higher powers. There is an obvious clinical implication here when advising a patient on the selection of a spectacle frame. At +1.00 DS, for example, a change in the boxed lens size of a frame from 52 mm to 54 mm will make very little difference in weight or thickness, but this will not be the same at higher powers.

Impact resistance

This topic is dealt with in more detail in Chapter 10. Essentially, plastics materials are inherently more impact resistant than glass, but the overall strength of a finished lens will depend on any surface treatment applied. It is essential in the USA to provide prescription spectacle lenses that are impact resistant to the Food and Drug Administration (FDA) standard. This standard requires that any lens must not break when impacted by a 15.9 mm steel ball weighing not less than 16 gm is dropped on the front surface from a height of not less than 1.27 m. In the UK, there is no drop ball requirement for general wear spectacles. However, BS EN ISO 14889 (1997) has a static load test for uncut lenses supplied in the European Community. In this test a 22-mm steel ball is placed on the uncut lens with a force of 100 N for 10 seconds.

Processing capability

One of the reasons why CR39 became such a popular lens material was its ease of processing and its ability to accept surface treatments. Any material that cannot be surfaced on conventional machinery is going to have an inherent disadvantage since it means that lenses cannot be stocked in semi-finished form, and the use of multifocal and varifocal lens forms involves centralized manufacture.

Plastics materials can have anti-scratch coatings applied, although no coating will bring the surface hardness of plastics materials up to that of glass, due to the inherently softer substrate to the material. Thus a very hard coating on a soft material will simply crack when stress is applied.

Plastics materials also score on their general ease of tinting compared with glass materials. In the 1960s, vacuum coating techniques were applied to enable thin-film tinted coatings to be applied to glass lenses. This was an advantage for manufacturers, since only white lenses needed to be stocked as opposed to a series of lenses with different solid tints. From the wearer's viewpoint, the lenses offered a tint density that was independent of prescription and a much wider range of colours and densities than had been available before; however, the tints were not always very reproducible. Plastics lenses in the form of CR39 offered even easier tinting with very simple apparatus (see Chapter 10).

Availability of lens materials

The choice of lens materials available today is almost bewildering in its complexity. A selection of some of the materials currently available is shown in Table 5.2. It is confusing that lens manufacturers do not always state whether their specifications are based on the 'd' or 'e' line for measurement of mean refractive index and constringence.

Glass lens material advances in recent years have included the availability of photochromic forms, which change density with incident light intensity in both crown glass and higher refractive index versions. Also, materials with high refractive index are now available up to a value of 1.9. At one time high-index lens materials in glass were all very heavy, but the production of satisfactory glass using titanium oxide as an index booster by Schott in the early 1970s revolutionized the technology.

Plastics materials have become available with steadily increasing refractive index. Generally these materials can be made thinner than CR39, as they are more rigid in form, although at the same time they can be less impact resistant. Polycarbonate has the highest impact resistance of any prescription lens material (Chapter 10).

Manufacture of lenses

The traditional manufacturing method for glass spectacle lenses was by a process known as *lapping*, where a block of glass is shaped by a metal tool (the lap) with the required curvature, the glass being removed by an abrasive slurry (Figure 5.6). The lapping tool moved from side to side about a vertical axis, in a pseudo-random pattern, and vertical pressure was applied to the surface being cut. Successively finer grades of abrasive produced a smoother surface, the final polishing being carried out by a felt pad stuck on to the cast iron tool.

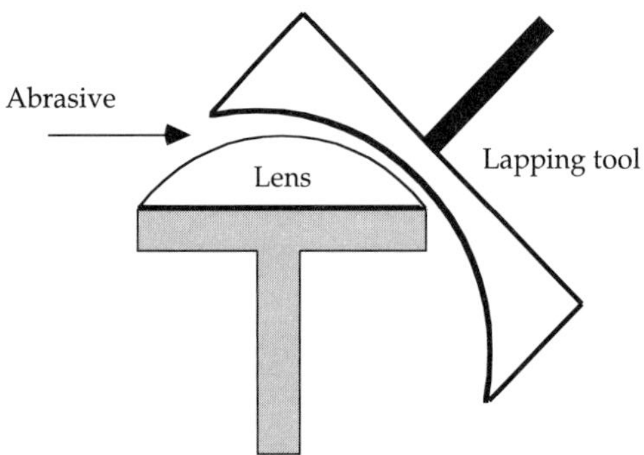

Figure 5.6. Lapping process for lens manufacture.

An unfortunate consequence of this process was that the tool abraded in time and had to be re-cut on a lap cutter in order to provide a true figure. Lapping is still extensively used in lens manufacture, but aluminium alloy tools are now commonly used, with interchangeable adhesive tool facings being used to provide the abrasion. Loose grinding medium is therefore no longer required, but a liquid coolant is still necessary for many materials. Thus the tool facing wears, but not the tool itself.

Although originally used on glass only, lapping also came to be used on CR39 material, and enabled laboratories to process this plastics material in a similar way to glass, except that different pressures and process times are required.

The initial production of a rough curve is slow by a lapping process, thus this stage is now carried out by *generation*. Figure 5.7 gives

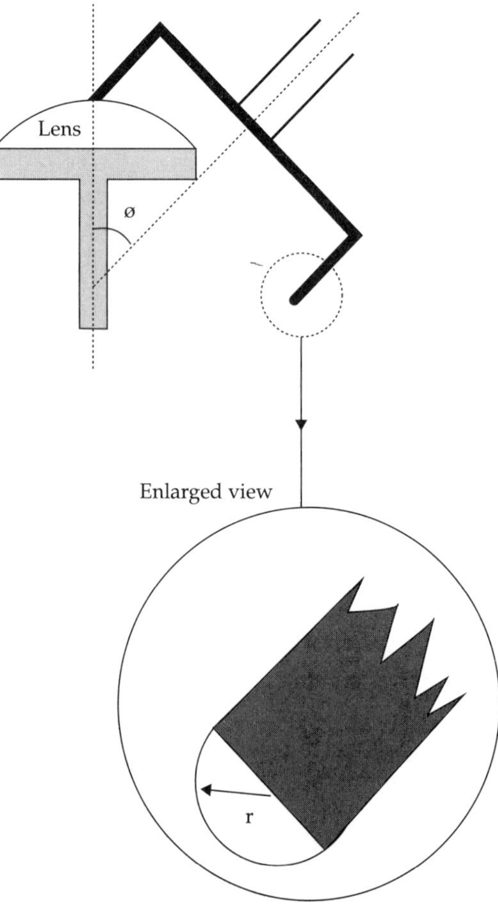

Figure 5.7. Universal spherical generator.

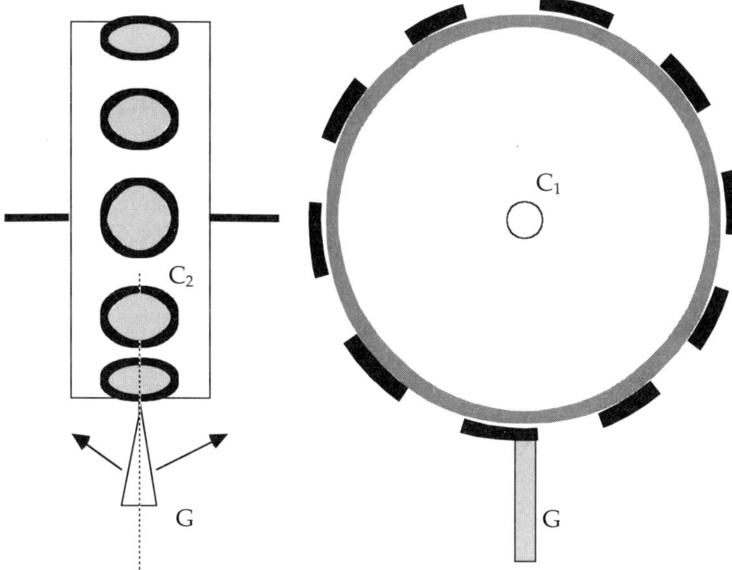

Figure 5.8. Mass production of convex toroidal surfaces on a toric wheel.

a diagrammatic representation of a crown tool with a radius of curvature of *r*, which has industrial diamond impregnated into the rim. This tool is presented at an angle of ϕ to the vertical.

The radius generated on the lens surface (r_c) is:

$$r_c = \frac{y}{\sin\phi}$$

where y is the semi diameter of the crown tool. As y is a constant for any tool, this means that the radius is inversely proportional to the sine of the angle of inclination, ϕ. This is the basis of the machine known as the *universal spherical generator*.

It is also possible to lap toroidal surfaces with toroidal tools; however, the geometry of the torus means that the tool and surface will only be in alignment along the equator of the torus. As the tool must move randomly across the surface in order to produce a fine figure, this means that true toroidal surfaces cannot be produced by lapping. However, it should be pointed out that the differences are very small indeed.

Just as spherical surfaces are no longer roughed by lapping but by generating, so now toroidal surfaces are also produced in this way. Different types of machinery are used for mass production and prescription work, the latter requiring equipment that can cut curves over a very wide range. Figure 5.8 shows equipment that was once used for the mass production of positive toroidal glass lens surfaces. A generator tool G abrades against lenses stuck around the outside of a wheel with centre of curvature C_1. The tool is also rotating about a second radius C_2, thus giving a surface with two different radii in perpendicular sections. If the two centres of curvature were made to coincide then spherical surfaces would be produced, but this is not the ideal form of manufacture. Smoothing and polishing machines can also be made in the same way. The radius of the wheel gives rise to the fixed *base curve* of the toroidal surface, and the position of C_2 can be varied to give various *cross curves*.

The geometry of the spherical generator can also be adapted to give the *universal toric generator*. Figures 5.9 and 5.10 illustrate the principles of this type of machine, which in its most comprehensive form can generate positive or negative surfaces. Some machines are limited to only generating negative power surfaces, and are mostly used for cutting prescription surfaces on multifocal and progressive lenses.

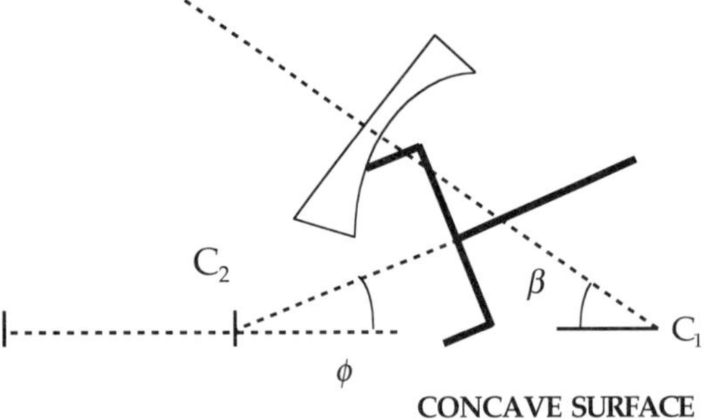

Figure 5.9. Schematic diagram of a universal toric generator, showing manufacture of negative surfaces.

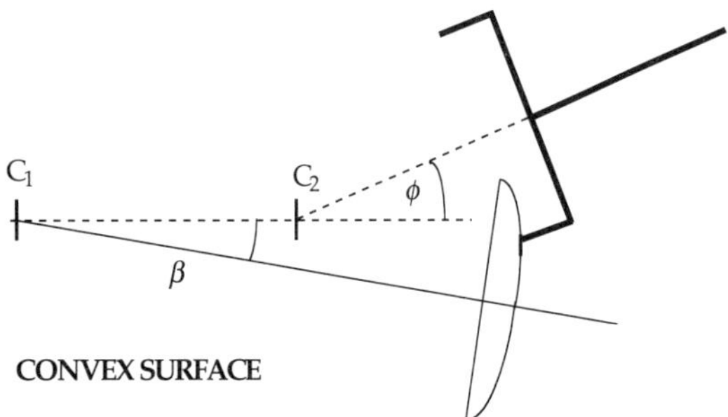

Figure 5.10. Schematic diagram of a universal toric generator, showing manufacture of positive surfaces.

Plastics lenses are mostly made in two different ways. Thermoplastic materials such as polymethyl methacrylate and polycarbonate are generally injection moulded, although polycarbonate is also dry cut on specially adapted toric generators.

CR39 and similar thermosetting materials are moulded from liquid monomer in glass moulds. Figure 5.11 shows the arrangement whereby front and rear glass moulds are separated by a flexible gasket. The gasket is essential to allow for the shrinkage of the plastics material during the polymerization process. The monomer and catalyst are injected into the space between the moulds, and then the whole assembly is heated. At one time it was normal to heat the lenses to between 40° and 80°C for around 16 hours. This could either be in an oven or a water bath. More recently much shorter cycles have been used, and some processes use ultraviolet radiation for the polymerization process.

After heat treatment to reduce internal stress (annealing), the gasket and moulds are

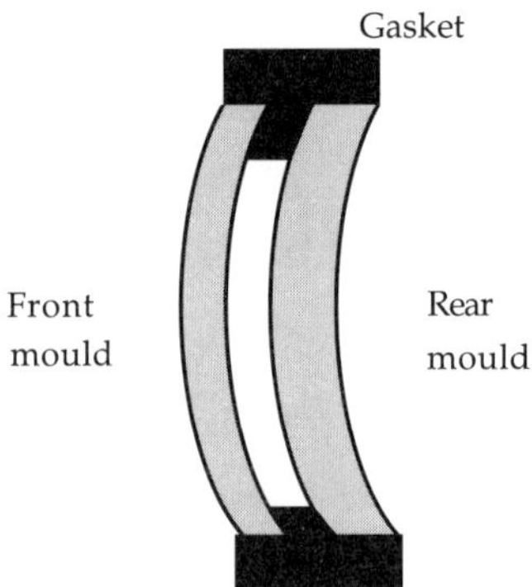

Figure 5.11. Process for manufacturing plastic lenses using glass moulds.

removed to give a finished lens. Because of the high level of internal stress in the process, the moulds used must be made of toughened glass.

Multifocal and progressive lens manufacture

The early development of multifocal and progressive lenses was very much limited by the available technology of production and lens materials. Split, cement and upcurve solid bifocals (see Chapter 8) can all be produced on the same machinery as single vision lenses. Fused bifocals also require relative simple surface processing, the complexity being in the heat fusing process that combines the segment glass with that of the major portion of the lens. Bubbles of air can be trapped between the two components, and if the heating is excessive the boundary between the two glass materials may become 'wavy'.

Downcurve solid bifocals in glass require specialist manufacturing equipment, as shown in Figure 5.12. Here the segment is manufactured at the centre of a large semi-finished lens, on the rear surface. The front surface of the lens is then worked spherical or toroidal as demanded by the prescription.

Progressive addition lenses have complex surfaces that are not generally rotationally symmetrical, so cannot be produced by grinding and polishing. Plastic lenses are produced from moulds, which are manufactured on numerically controlled milling machines.

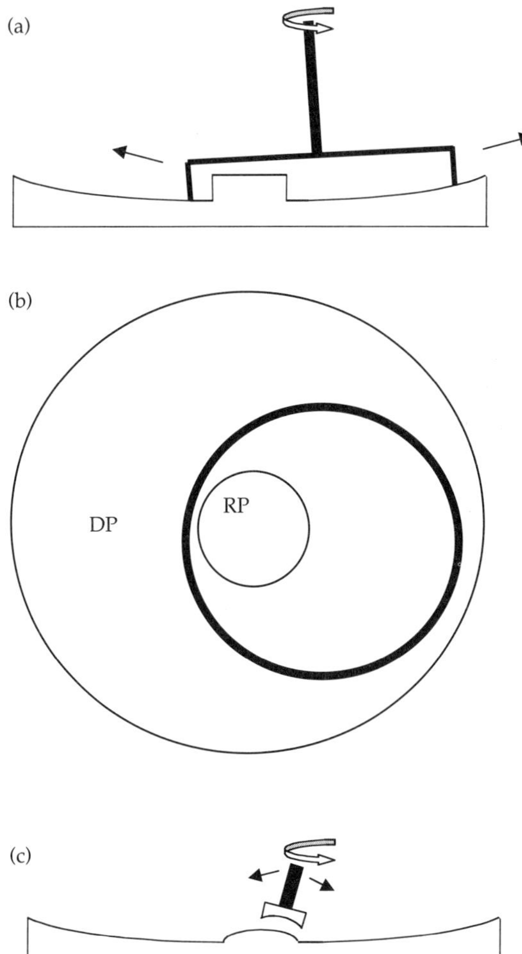

Figure 5.12. Manufacture of downcurve solid glass bifocals. (a) Annular crown generating tool used to leave a central segment area (b). (c) Small segment generating tool.

Glass lenses are traditionally formed by a process called 'slumping', where glass is allowed to soften and sag on to a ceramic block. The ceramic blocks are also produced by numerically controlled milling machines but, unlike the plastic moulds, allowance has to be made for the thickness of glass used (Figure 5.13).

For many years the supply of multifocals and progressive addition lenses has been a multi-stage process. The lenses are produced in semi-finished form with just the segment (or progressive) side finished. These are then distributed to laboratories or to opticians with their own manufacturing facilities, where the

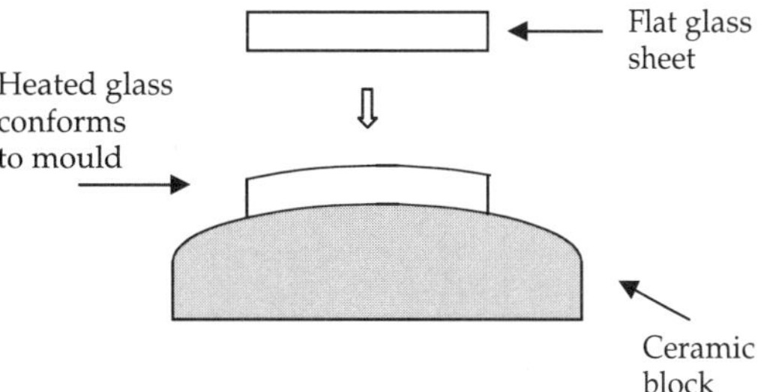

Figure 5.13. Glass 'slumping' process for the manufacture of progressive addition lens surfaces.

second surface is processed to comply with a specific prescription (Figure 5.14).

The demand for rapid supply of spectacle lenses to prescription has caused some novel manufacturing techniques to be developed. Although finished single vision uncut lenses can be supplied from stock and rapidly edged to the required shape, the same is not true of multifocal and progressive lenses. With these lenses there are too many variables to stock finished forms. One method is to use a small scale CR39 casting unit, where a suitable front surface containing an addition is combined with an appropriate rear surface mould which has a spherical or toroidal component as demanded by the prescription.

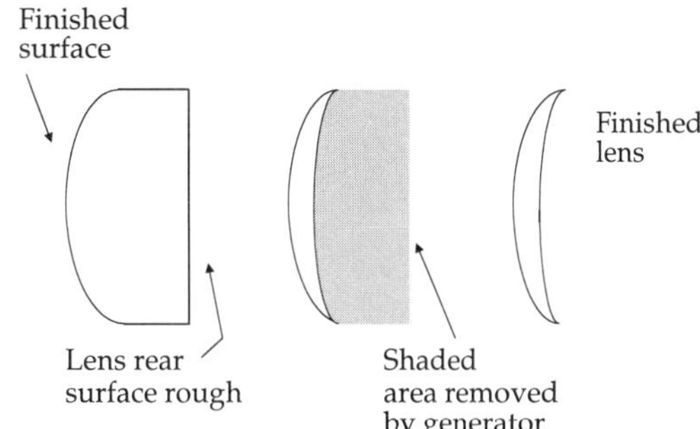

Figure 5.14. Manufacture of lenses from the semi-finished state.

Another method for rapid manufacture of multifocals and progressives is to use a combination of thin wafers, the front one containing the addition, the rear one the cylinder, which are cemented together by a rapidly curing adhesive. This process can be used to manufacture both glass and plastics lenses (Figure 5.15).

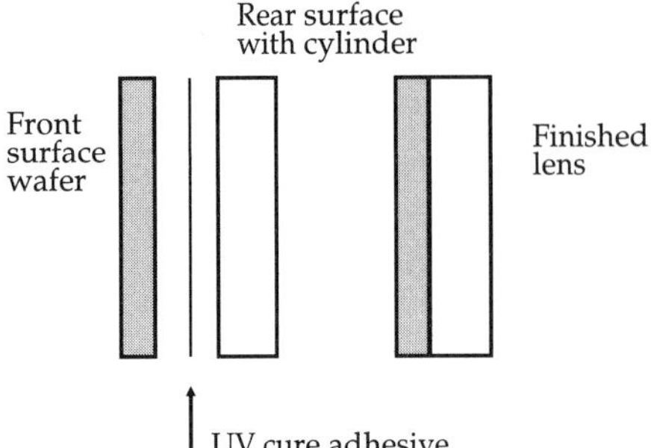

Figure 5.15. Manufacture of lenses from wafer elements.

Lens edging

After the lens has been finished on both surfaces, it is then described as an *uncut*. The next process is cutting this uncut to the required shape to fit in to a specific spectacle frame. Originally this process was carried out by hand, using a water-cooled stone edging wheel. However, automatic machinery is now almost exclusively used, the required shape being cut from the uncut either by copying a plastic template of the lens shape or by storing the shape electronically in the machine after scanning the spectacle frame with a mechanical or optical sensor. Some hand finishing of the lens may be necessary, for example to remove sharp edges on negative power lenses.

Summary

This chapter discusses the properties of glass and plastic lens materials, and describes some of the processes used for the manufacture of single vision, multifocal and progressive addition lenses.

6

Measurement of lens power

Introduction

Assessment of lens power is a fundamental requirement for any person dealing with spectacle lenses. Whether checking the power of a newly glazed pair of spectacles prior to final collection or determining the specification of an unknown pair of lenses, a quick and accurate method is essential.

As described in this Chapter, two methods for determining vertex powers are readily available – neutralization by known-power lenses, and measurement on a focimeter. The first of these techniques requires no more instrumentation than a set of trial case lenses, but is considered obsolete by many. However, neutralization is still extensively taught on many ophthalmic courses as it provides a valuable grounding in basic concepts of spectacle lenses. Focimeters, the method of choice in most settings, have become sophisticated instruments, with many fully automatic versions available.

Neutralization

The principle of neutralization is that an unknown-power spectacle lens is combined with a known-power trial-case lens in order to provide a combination with zero power, the known-power lens thus neutralizing the unknown lens. The technique is straightforward in the case of spherical power lenses, but can appear less straightforward for cylindrical power lenses.

The reason why neutralization works well is in the method used for determining the neutral point of the combination. The method uses the visual detection of image movement, and can best be explained diagrammatically. In Figure 6.1a, a positive lens is shown simplified into two plane prisms mounted base to base. If this 'lens' is moved, then, as shown in

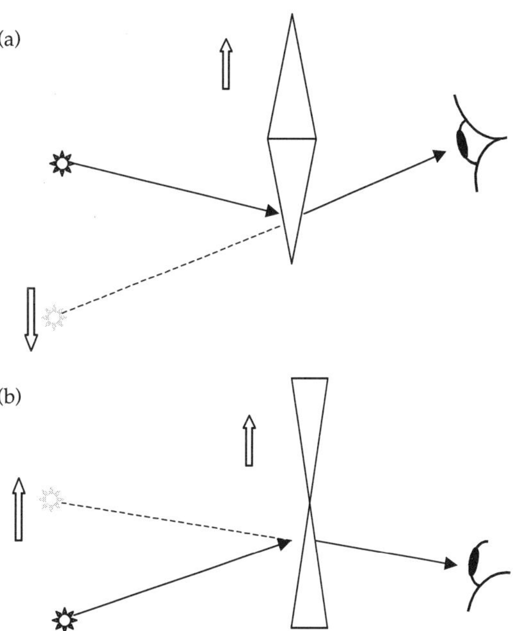

Figure 6.1. Schematic diagram of transverse movements in neutralization. (a) Positive power lens, simulated by two prisms mounted base to base. (b) Negative power lens simulated by two prisms mounted apex to apex.

the figure, the image will appear to move towards the prism apex, in the opposite direction to the lens movement (an 'against' movement). The image movement is called a *transverse image movement*. Conversely, as shown in Figure 6.1b, a negative power lens will give movement of the image in the same direction as the lens movement (a 'with' movement). If the lens has no power, or the combination of the unknown lens and the known-power lens has no power, then movements of the lens give no movement of the image. The technique is very sensitive to residual power errors, so that powers of 0.25 D can be detected.

In the case of lenses having cylindrical power, a similar analogy can be used to explain the image movements seen when a lens is rotated in plan view. Figure 6.2 shows a positive power cylinder consisting of two plano prisms mounted base to base. Note that as the lens is rotated clockwise, the prism deviates the image towards the apex on each side. The rotational movement observed is called a *'scissors' movement*.

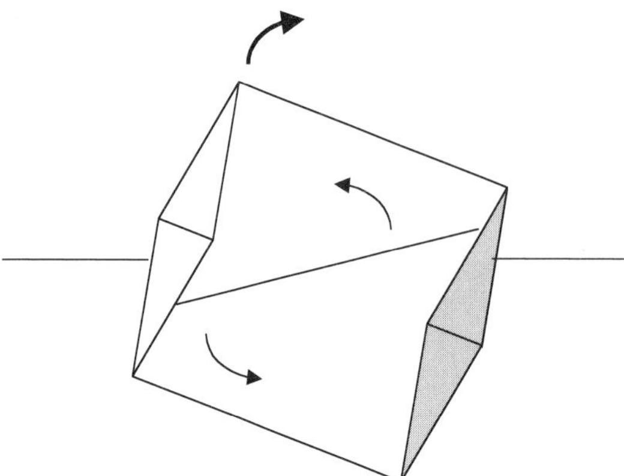

Figure 6.2. Rotational movement of the image in a positive cylinder, simulated by two prisms mounted base to base.

(a)

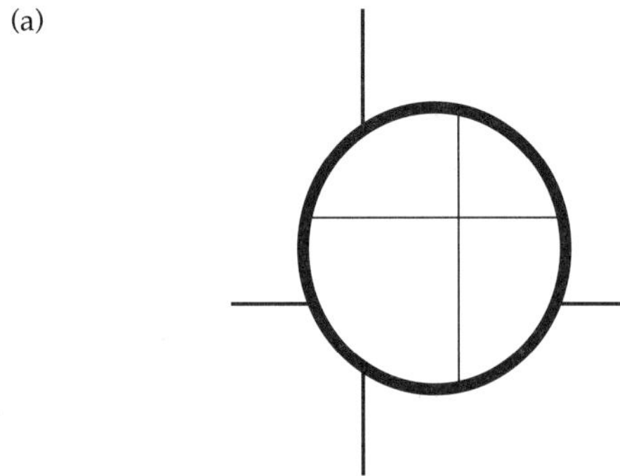

(b)

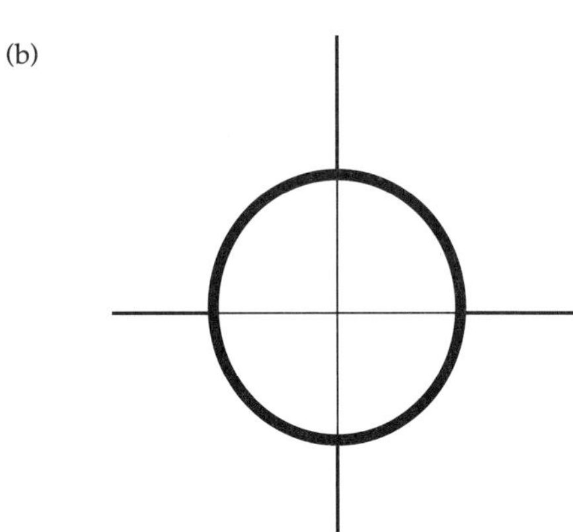

Figure 6.3. Determination of the optical centre in neutralization. In (a), the optical centre of the lens is not coincident with the centre of the target and the image is displaced due to prismatic effects (Chapter 4). In (b), the optical centre is coincident with the centre of the cross target and the image of the cross is undeviated in position.

Procedure for neutralization of spherical power lenses

1. Mark the optical centre of the unknown lens. The optical centre is the point on the lens through which light passes undeviated (see Chapter 1). To find the optical centre, use a cross target and position the lens so that the image of the cross is coincident with the object (Figure 6.3). Dot on the lens with a pen at the point where the vertical and horizontal lines intersect.
2. View a near target and determine whether the lens is positive or negative, depending on the image movement in relation to the lens movement. A positive lens gives an 'against' movement, and a negative lens gives a 'with' movement.
3. Using lenses of opposite power to the unknown lens, determine the value of the neutralizing lens. Therefore, if a 'with' movement is seen positive lenses should be added, whilst if an 'against' movement is observed negative lenses should be used to neutralize the movement. The lenses must be held in contact (see Figure 6.4), with the neutralizing lenses held coaxial to the

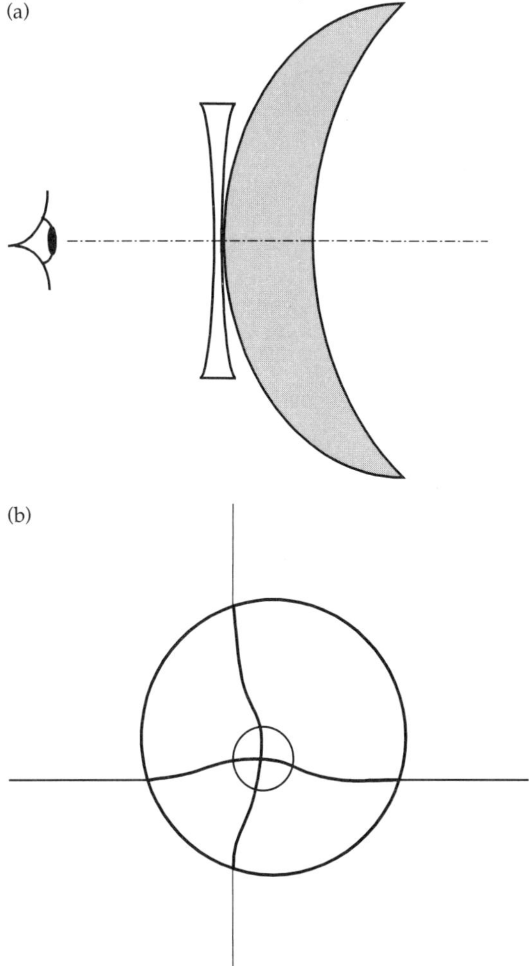

Figure 6.4. (a) Arrangement of lenses for neutralization, with the trial lens held against the front surface of the spectacle lens. Note the air gap at the edge of the trial lens. (b) Poor image of a target as seen through a high power lens and neutralizing lens, where an air gap gives variable neutralization. An aperture should be used to restrict the view to the central circle.

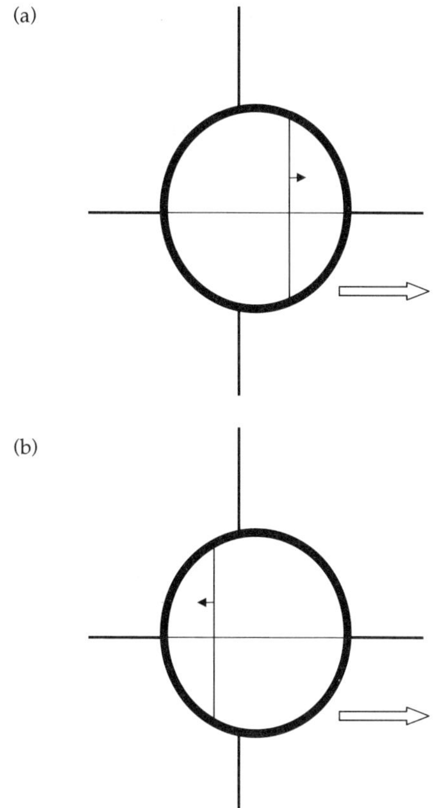

Figure 6.5. Neutralizing movements. In (a), a negative power lens is moved to the right. The vertical image moves in the same direction, known as a 'with' movement. In (b), a positive power lens is moved to the right, with the image of a vertical line moving in the opposite direction. This is known as an 'against' movement.

optical centre of the unknown lens. The most efficient way to determine the neutral point is to use a 'bracketing' technique. For example, if the initial movement observed is a 'with' movement, use a moderately powered positive trial lens (e.g. +4.00 DS) as the first lens of choice. Assuming that the combination of lenses now gives an 'against' movement, split the difference between the first two trial lenses used (i.e. zero and +4.00 DS) and use a +2.00 DS trial lens. Continue 'splitting the difference' between trial lenses giving 'with' and 'against' movements until the neutral point has been bracketed to the nearest 0.25 DS. A bracketing method is much more efficient than starting with a low-powered trial lens and working up the trial case until the movement is neutralized.

4. Write down the power of the neutralizing lens, but with the opposite sign, as the power of the unknown lens.

For the neutralization technique to work accurately, the following points must be observed:

1. The unknown lens and the neutralizing lens(es) should be in contact. In view of the diameter of neutralizing lenses and the meniscus form of most present-day

spectacle lenses, this means that the neutralizing lens must be held against the front surface of the spectacle lens (Figure 6.4). This means in turn that the eventual power determined is the front vertex power, whereas normally spectacle lenses are described in terms of their back vertex power (Chapter 1). Unless the lens is very thick, the difference between the two values will be minimal compared to the observer's errors. At one time, lenses in special mounts with a small effective diameter were manufactured by Stigmat specifically for neutralizing the BVP of a curved form lens. However, this development was rendered obsolete by the production of low cost focimeters.

2. Care must be taken with positive power lenses that a magnified, erect image is being viewed. As shown in Figure 6.6a, it is possible for a strong positive lens to produce an inverted image between the lens and the observer if the object viewed is too far away from the lens. The theory of neutralization relies on the viewing of virtual images, as shown for positive and negative lenses in Figure 6.6b and c respectively. Thus, to avoid the situation in Figure 6.6a, a near object should be used during the initial stages of neutralization.

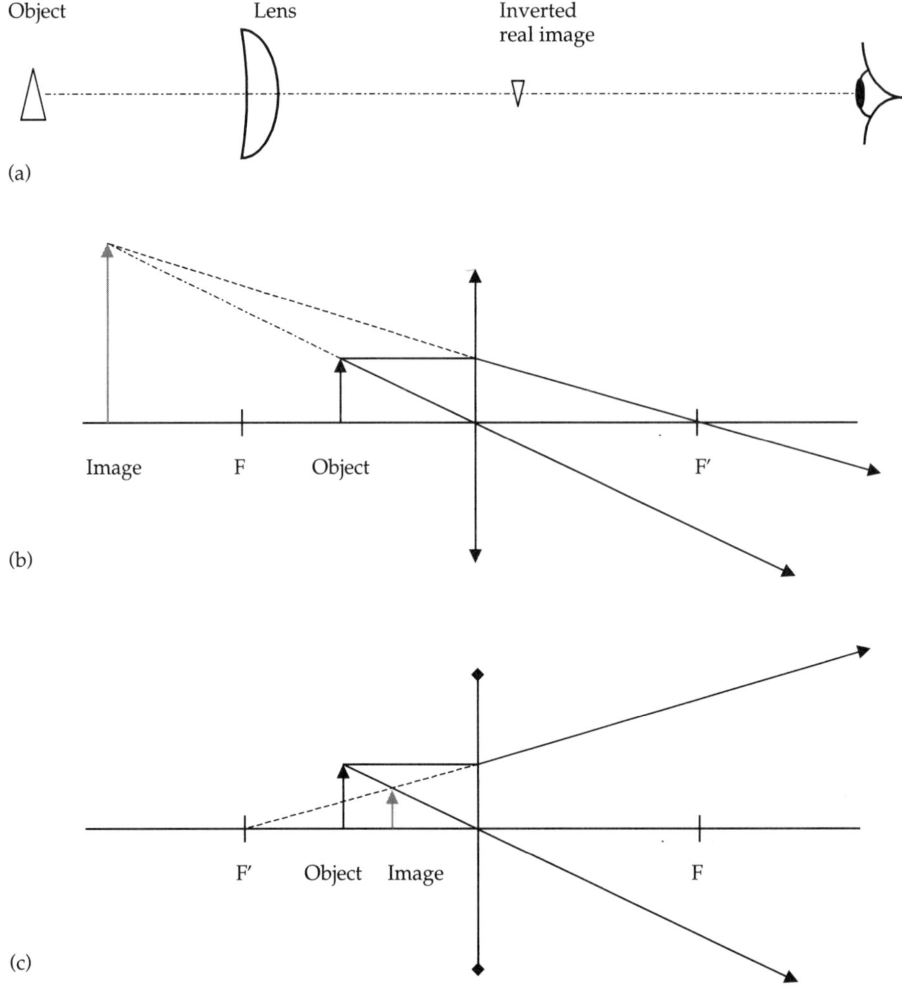

Figure 6.6. Formation of images during neutralization. (a) A positive lens viewing a distant target, resulting in a real, inverted image. (b) A positive lens viewing a near object, resulting in a virtual, erect image. (c) A negative lens viewing a near object, resulting in a virtual, erect image.

3. During the final stages of neutralization, a target should be used that is as far away as possible, and the lenses held at arm's length. These conditions give the most sensitivity in determining the end point of neutralization.
4. With high power lenses, particularly positive power lenses, it is difficult to neutralize across the whole of the trial lens aperture due to the variable air gap away from the optical centre. Thus a small paper aperture can be introduced over the unknown lens, centred on the optical centre, in order to confine the view to the central portion only (Figure 6.4b).

Procedure for neutralization of cylindrical power lenses

Cylindrical power lenses can be identified by the *rotation test*. View a straight-line target and rotate the lens in plan view. If the lens is spherical, then there will be no change in angular position of the image relative to the object. However, in the case of a cylindrical or sphero-cylindrical power lens, the image will rotate, the direction depending on the power and orientation of the cylinder (Figure 6.7). The amount of rotation depends on the size of the cylinder, being more marked for higher cylinder powers. The rotation test can also be used to determine the cylindrical axis, since when the axis of the cylinder and the object are parallel, there will be no angular deviation of the image.

1. Mark the optical centre and cylindrical axes by finding the position in which the lens can be held over a target without introducing rotational movement. Note by marking on the lens whether the marked axis is the more positive or the more negative. This notation is relative rather than absolute; there will not always be one positive and one negative meridian, but one will always be more positive than the other. Both axes should pass through the optical centre.
2. Holding the lens with the cylinder axis parallel to the target, move the lens transversely (i.e. perpendicular to the cylinder axis) and neutralize the movement with spherical lenses.

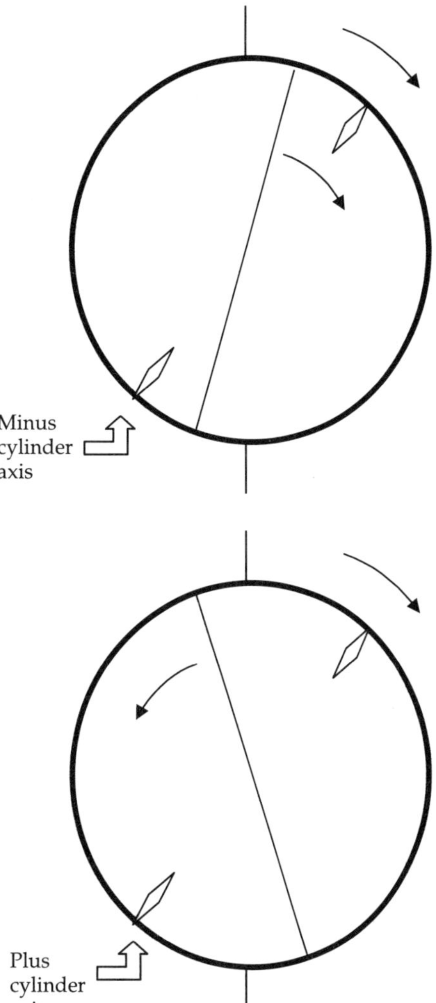

Figure 6.7. Rotational image movements from cylindrical lenses. (a) A negative power cylinder produces a 'with' image rotation in the same direction as the lens. (b) A positive power cylinder gives an 'against' rotation of the image in the opposite direction to the lens.

3. Turn the lens through 90° and neutralize the second meridian.
4. Measure the axes. Place the lens, front surface uppermost, on a lens protractor with the horizontal of the lens parallel to the 0–180 line of the protractor (Figure 6.8). The optical centre should be over the centre of the protractor. Read off the angle of the axis marking, taking care to read from the correct scale on the protractor.
5. Write down the two lens powers found in point (2) above, *but with the opposite sign*, in

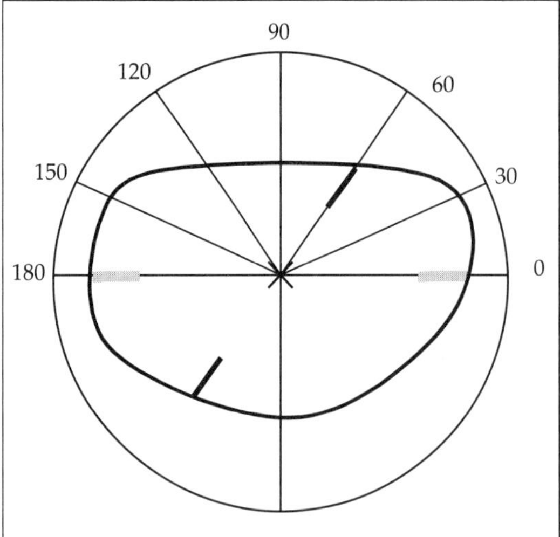

Figure 6.8. Standard axis notation for cylindrical lenses. The diagram shows a lens with an axis of 60° being measured, the optical centre of the lens having been placed on the centre of the protractor. Note that a large scale interval has been used on the protractor for clarity.

order to give the actual power of the lens. Note whether the measured axis is positive or negative. For example, if the neutralizing lenses were +2.00 D and +3.00 D, the actual lens powers will be –2.00 D and –3.00 D. In this case, the 'more positive' meridian would have been the –2.00 D meridian. If the positive cylinder axis is at 35, then the prescription can be immediately deduced as:

–2.00 DC × 35/–3.00 DC × 125
(cross-cylinder form)

The prescription is written in this form since –2.00 is the more positive power, and is therefore associated with the positive axis. The other axis must therefore be 125, as principal meridians are always mutually perpendicular.

6. The prescription in point (5) can then be converted by transposition (Chapter 3) to either of the sphero-cylindrical forms as required:

   –2.00 DS/–1.00 DC × 125 or
   –3.00 DS/+1.00 DC × 35

In the procedure described above, the lens prescription is derived in cross-cylinder form by neutralizing each meridian separately with spherical trial lenses. If required, the result can then be transposed into sphero-cylindrical format. An alternative procedure is to neutralize the lens directly in sphero-cylindrical format, as follows:

1. Identify and mark the axes of the principle meridians.
2. Neutralize one meridian with a spherical lens, as before.
3. *Leaving the spherical lens in place,* examine the movement for the other principle meridian. Neutralize this movement using a cylindrical trial lens placed with its axis parallel to the target being viewed, and perpendicular to the direction of movement. For example, if the target being viewed is horizontal, the transverse lens movement will be vertical, and the cyl axis should be placed horizontally.
4. Measure the cylinder axis in the same way as before.
5. Write down the powers of the lenses used in sphero-cylindrical format. Remember to reverse the sign of the neutralizing lenses, but write down the cylinder axis as you have found it. For example, the neutralizing lenses may have been +2.00 DS, and +1.00 DC at an axis that is measured on the protractor as being 125. The prescription is therefore –2.00 DS/–1.00 DC × 125.
6. If the answer is required in positive sphero-cylindrical form, the more negative meridian should be neutralized first with the sphere. Conversely, if a negative sphero-cylindrical format is required, the more positive meridian should be neutralized first.

Neutralization of prism

Prism can also be readily neutralized by hand. A lens incorporating a prism can be identified by comparing the position of the optical centre of the lens to that of a specified centration point, such as the boxed centre of the lens (Chapter 4). If the two points are not coincident, then the lens has a prismatic effect at the centration point. In many cases, the optical centre will not be on the lens at all. The base–apex direction of an unknown prism is identified since a prism deviates light towards its apex (Figure 6.9a). Having identified the orientation of the prism,

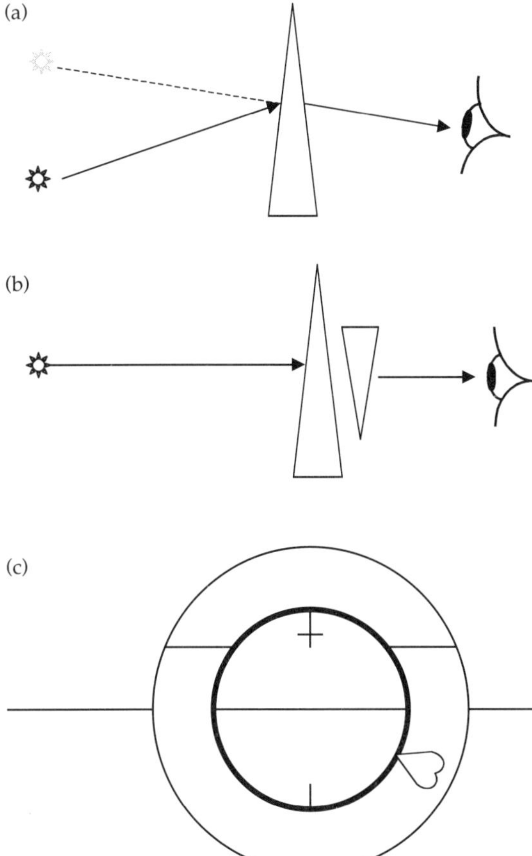

Figure 6.9. (a) Deviation of light towards the apex by a prismatic lens. (b) Schematic arrangement for the neutralization of prisms. In practice, the lenses would be in contact. (c) Neutralization of image deviation by using prism of equal power and opposite base setting.

it can be neutralized by holding a prism of known power with base–apex direction opposite to that of the unknown prism (Figure 6.9b). The prism is neutralized when the known-power prism eliminates the deviation at the centration point (Figure 6.9c).

An alternative method to determine the power of a prism is to use a tangent scale. We know that prismatic power, $P = 100 \tan d$ (Equation 1.11). So, if a prism of 1Δ is held 1 m from a screen, the deviation at the screen will be 1 cm. Likewise, if the 1Δ prism is held 2 m from the screen, the deviation produced will be 2 cm, and so on. Therefore, a scale can be produced with graduations in centimetres equivalent to the working distance in metres. To use the scale, the prism should be orientated

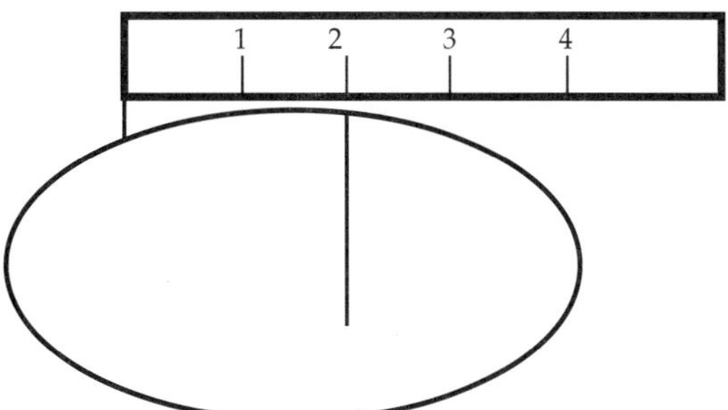

Figure 6.10. Tangent scale. Lens is held at the correct distance from the scale. The base of the prism is to the left, and the image of the scale zero marking has been moved coincident with the 2Δ marking.

so that the observer looks through the boxed centre towards the line representing zero on the scale, and the apex of the prism is pointing onto the scale (Figure 6.10). The image will be deviated by the prism towards its apex, and the point on the scale to which the zero line is deviated gives the prismatic power in prism dioptres.

Neutralization of near addition

To neutralize a near vision segment in a multifocal lens (bifocal or trifocal), use the same procedure as for the distance prescription, and note that the axes will be the same as those found for the distance. The difference between the spherical distance and near powers gives the power of the addition. For example:

Distance	*Near*	*Addition*
+1.00 DS	+3.00 DS	+2.00 DS
–3.00 DS/–0.50 DC × 170	–1.50 DS/–0.50 DC × 170	+1.50 DS

The optical centre of the addition, considered as a separate lens, will be at the centre of the segment. However, the position of the near optical centre will depend on the characteristics of the distance lens and the near addition in combination (see Chapter 8). It is quite easy to find lenses where the near optical centre is not on the lens at all, even though there is no prescribed prism. Therefore, do not mark the near optical centre or try to neutralize prism at near for 'invisible' bifocals.

The focimeter

The focimeter is now the commonest instrument in use for the measurement of lens power, and is available in several different forms.

Visually focusing instruments

A ray diagram of a typical arrangement of an eyepiece focusing focimeter is shown in Figure 6.11. An illuminated target (T) moves longitudinally along the optic axis of the instrument, and is connected to a power scale (S) reading vertex lens power in dioptres. The unknown spectacle lens is placed on a holder (L) at the second principal focus of the positive collimating lens (C). The purpose of this design feature, which is an example of a Badal lens system, is to ensure that the magnification of the focimeter image remains constant regardless of the power of the unknown spectacle lens: the spectacle lens is said to be in the 'unit magnification' position. The astronomical telescope, consisting of an objective (O) and an eyepiece (E), is adjusted so that it is focused on infinity, and therefore only parallel light will be seen in focus. The graticule (G) in the eyepiece of the telescope contains axis and prism scales. Note that a narrow band-pass filter (F) is used to provide a peak illumination at either 546.07 nm or 587.56 nm.

In Figure 6.11, the instrument is shown at zero adjustment with no spectacle lens in place. Light emerges from the collimating lens system in parallel, and the image seen through the telescope is sharp with the target positioned at zero on the power scale, where the target is coincident with the first principle focus of the collimating lens. In Figure 6.12a, a positive power spectacle lens has been introduced at the lens holder (L). The target has been moved closer to the collimating lens by a distance x in order that parallel light leaves the front of the spectacle lens and is seen in focus by the telescope. The image of the target is situated at a distance x' from the rear surface of the unknown spectacle lens. In Figure 6.12b, the alternative situation with a negative power spectacle lens is shown. In this case, the target has been moved further away from the unknown lens, by a distance x, in order to be seen in focus by the telescope. The distance x' again gives the distance from the rear lens surface to the image focus.

The relationship of target movement to the power of the unknown lens can be deduced from Newton's relationship:

$$f^2 = -x.x' \qquad \textit{Equation 6.01}$$

As x' is the back vertex focal length of the lens being measured, this means that the target movement per dioptre (x) is proportional to the back vertex power of the lens, and that

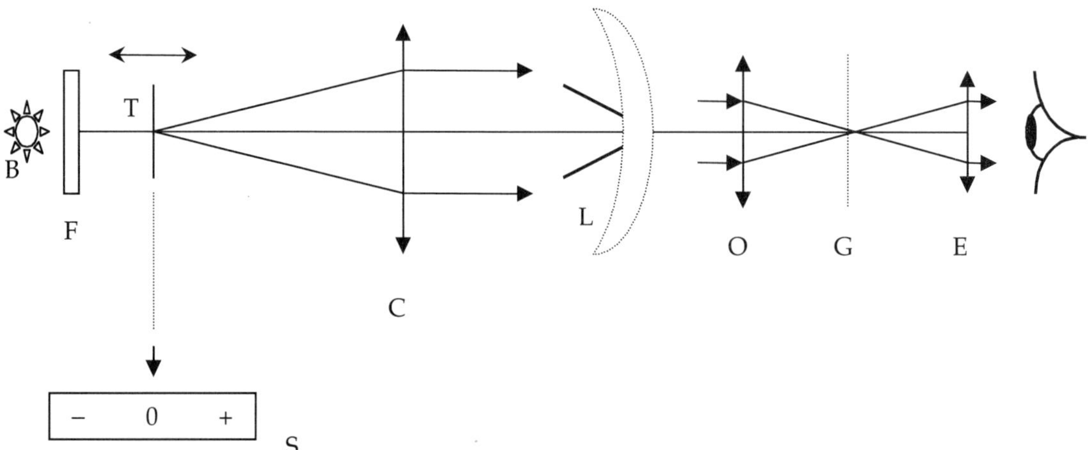

Figure 6.11. Ray diagram of an eyepiece focimeter, with no unknown lens in place. Light from a bulb (B) is filtered (F) and illuminates a target (T) connected to a power scale (S). The collimating lens (C) is placed one focal length from the zeroed target, and a lens rest (L) is placed one focal length from the collimating lens. Light emerging from the system enters a telescope consisting of an objective (O), an eyepiece (E) and a graticule (G).

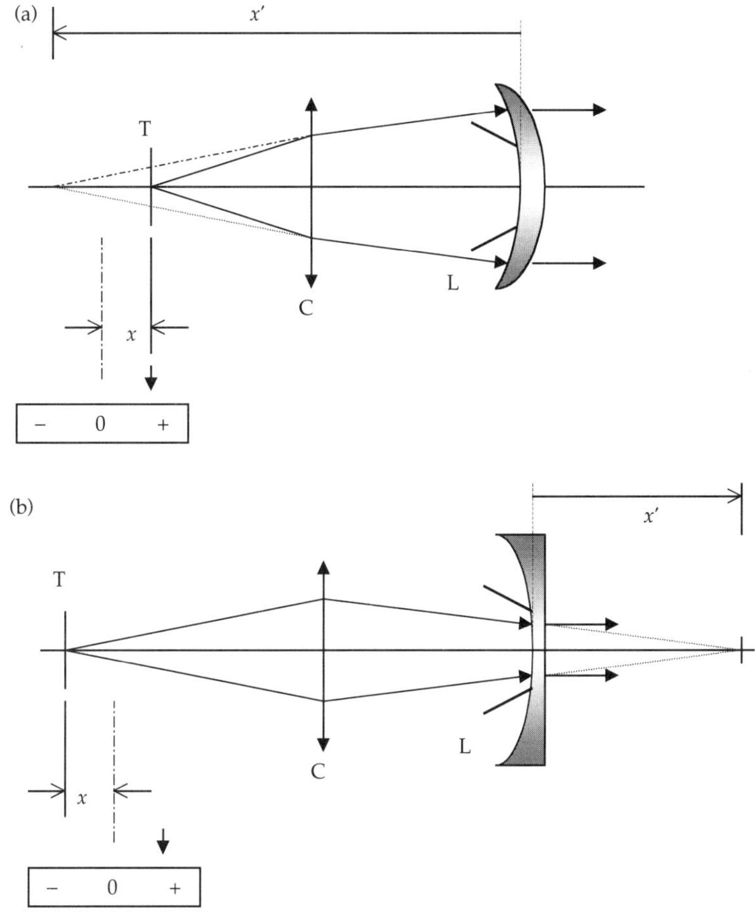

Figure 6.12. A focimeter with (a) a positive spectacle lens in place, and (b) a negative lens in place.

the focimeter power scale is linear. f is the focal length of the collimating lens, sometimes known as the 'standard' lens of a focimeter.

The selection of collimating lens power is a compromise between the range, accuracy, and dimensions of the instrument. Equation 6.1 above can be rearranged to give the target movement (in mm) per dioptre of unknown lens power:

$$x = \frac{1000}{F^2} \qquad \textit{Equation 6.02}$$

where F is the power of the collimating lens in dioptres. For a collimating lens power of +25 D, the target movement is 1.6 mm/D. This demands a very precise calibration and control of target movement in order to obtain accurate results; however, on the other hand, in order to measure over a range of +10 D to –10 D, a target movement of only 32 mm is required. If as an alternative design a collimating lens power of +10 D were to be used, this would give a target movement of 10 mm/D and a total target movement of 200 mm, giving a very large but theoretically more accurate instrument.

In order to obtain accurate results from a visually focusing eyepiece instrument (Figure 6.13), the instrument must first have the eyepiece adjusted to minimize any proximal accommodation. Proximal accommodation is induced when the eye looks into an instrument that is focused for infinity and thus requires no accommodation. However, the viewer is aware that the instrument is of finite length and accommodation is stimulated. The procedure for

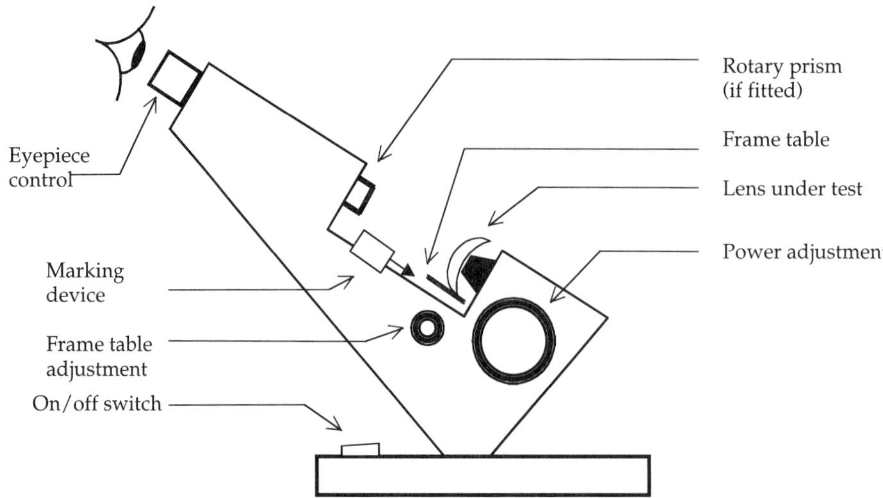

Figure 6.13. Line diagram of the major components of the focimeter.

correcting for proximal accommodation is as follows:

1. Before inserting an unknown lens into the focimeter, set the target position at zero by means of the power drum control.
2. Unscrew the eyepiece adjustment control until the target goes completely out of focus.
3. Screw in the eyepiece control until the target just comes into focus. The graticule should also be in focus at the same time.
4. Check by setting the power control drum to a random value and then visually refocusing the target; the value on the power control should read zero.

Note that if the target and graticule cannot be made to appear jointly in focus at zero indicated power, then a more fundamental adjustment is required by an instrument mechanic.

In order to overcome some of the above potential problems when using eyepiece focimeters, instruments known as projection focimeters have been developed. In these the image is projected on to a translucent screen, which is optically coincident with the plane of the graticule. It is also claimed that projection instruments are less tiring to use over a long period of time than those with eyepieces.

Although the majority of visually focusing instruments use continuously indicating analogue scales, which require interpolation between scale markings, some models use electronic digital displays, which can be adjusted to round off the reading to the nearest 0.12 or 0.25 D.

Basic use of the focimeter

Several different designs of illuminated target are used in focimeters. The simplest of these is the circle of dots or corona target (Figure 6.14). The spectacles or lens to be measured should be placed, rear surface down, on the aperture of the focimeter so as to measure

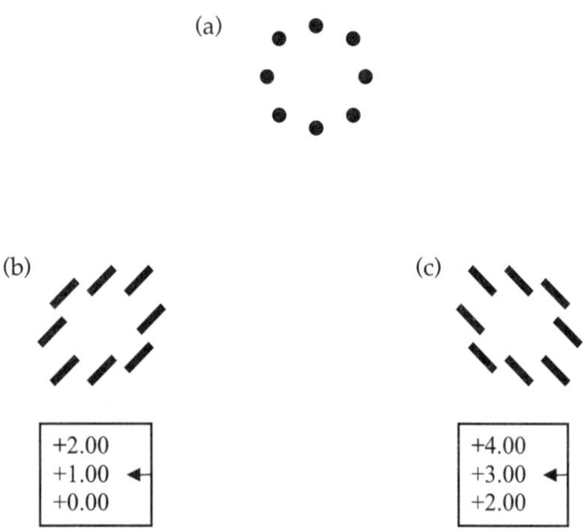

Figure 6.14. (a) Corona focimeter target. (b) Images of target seen when +1.00/+2.00 × 135 is focused first on the axis 45 image (b), and secondly on the axis 135 image (c), with associated power readings.

back vertex power as opposed to front vertex power. The lens should be positioned so that the boxed centre or other appropriate reference point is over the centre of the aperture and the lens is supported by the frame table.

The frame table is an adjustable support that enables a horizontal reference to be found for a pair of spectacles. The height is adjustable so that the optical axis can be positioned vertically at the required height. It is important for finding the cylinder axis accurately that both lens rims of a pair of spectacles being measured rest on the frame table.

A lens-marking device is normally provided which marks three ink dots on the front surface of the lens. The central dot is coincident with the optical axis of the instrument, and a line through all three dots is coincident with the 0–180 line on the axis scale of the protractor. This line should also be parallel to the frame table.

A spherical lens will give an image the same as the object – that is, the power wheel should be adjusted until the corona is again sharp, and the lens power read off from the scale.

Although not a standard accessory, an accessory 'dotting lens' would be very useful if supplied with visually focusing focimeters. The 'dotting lens' was suggested by Davis (1979) and consists of an annular positive lens, which converts the periphery of the focimeter telescope into a long focus microscope. This enables the front surface of the lens to be viewed at the same time as the focimeter image, thus a mark on the front of the lens can be aligned very accurately with the axis of the focimeter. This is useful in progressive addition lenses, for example, where prism is measured at a point marked on the lens by the manufacturer (Chapter 9).

Measurement of cylindrical power

In the case of an astigmatic lens the image will be distorted into a series of lines, rather than appearing as a ring of dots. Since all astigmatic lenses form two images with mutually perpendicular orientations, two positions of focus can be found (Figure 6.14). In order to determine the cylindrical axis, a marker on the graticule is generally made rotatable so that it can be made parallel with the clearest image line, and the axis can be read off the graticule protractor. The length of the line images in a corona target focimeter depends on the difference in power between the two meridians; the greater the power of the cylinder, the longer the line images that are formed.

In order to make a focimeter more accurate at determining the power of low power cylindrical lenses, targets are sometimes used which contain a line or series of lines (Figure 6.15). The lines can be used at any orientation with a spherical lens, but in order to obtain a clear focus with an astigmatic lens the target must first be orientated parallel to the

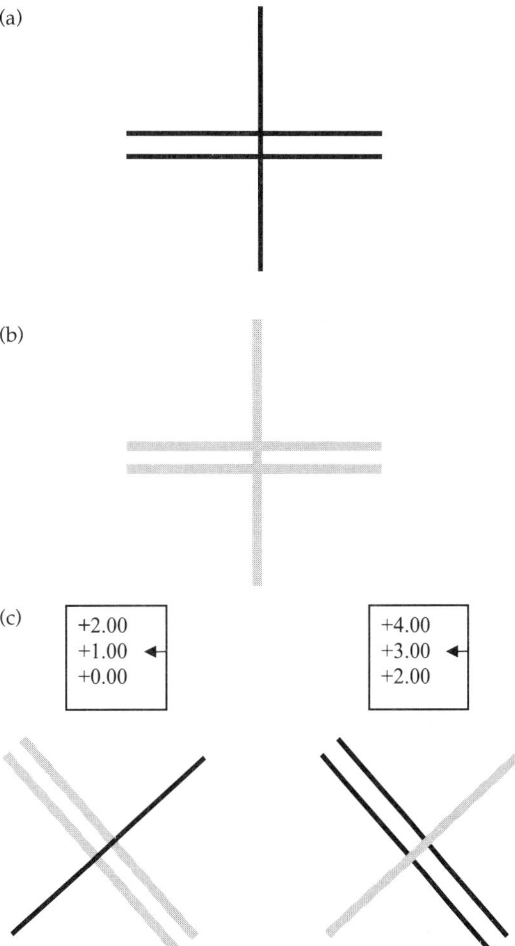

Figure 6.15. (a) Line focimeter target. (b) Blurred image due to target not being orientated parallel to the principal meridians of the lens. (c) Target correctly orientated, viewing the principal lens powers of +1.00/+2.00 × 135.

relevant principal meridian. The target orientation control is often calibrated in standard notation, and can be used as a cross check to the axis finder in the graticule for determining the axis of the cylinder. The target orientation control is particularly useful when it is impractical to position the focimeter image in the centre of the graticule, for example when measuring the near addition in multifocals.

A standard visually focusing focimeter does not measure cylindrical power directly. The two principal powers are measured, with their axes, giving a prescription in cross-cylinder form. For example, the powers and axes read off on the focimeter could be:

+5.25 DC × 90/+6.00 DC × 180

Which is equivalent to:

+5.25 DS/+0.75 DC × 180 or
+6.00 DS/–0.75 DC × 90

in sphero-cylindrical form.

Some focimeters with digital indication of power can produce the sphero-cylindrical form directly.

Measurement of prism

A very useful feature of all focimeters is their ability to measure prism (Chapter 4). When the focimeter image is over the centre of the graticule, the optical centre of the lens is over the lens clamp aperture. Deviation of the image from this point indicates the prismatic effect. The graticule of the focimeter is calibrated in prism dioptres so that the prismatic effect at any point on a lens can be read off. Note, however, that image displacement is in the direction of the *base* of the prism, which is the opposite to the situation in normal viewing, where the image is displaced towards the apex of the prism. In the focimeter, the astronomical telescope reverses the image position. The prismatic effect of the lens in Figure 6.16 is 2Δ Base Up and 2Δ horizontally (In or Out depending on whether it is a left or right lens respectively).

Owing to the limitations of the field of view through the instrument, most focimeters are limited to direct prism measurements of around 6Δ. A useful accessory on the focimeter is a variable power or rotary prism, fitted to the end of the telescope, which typically adds 15Δ of extra prism measuring range. The extra range is particularly useful when measuring the near power through a multifocal lens with high distance power.

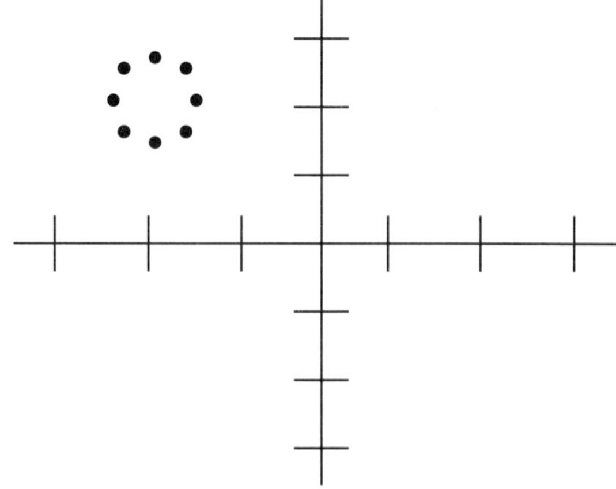

Figure 6.16. View into a focimeter eyepiece with a line target, where the lens incorporates 2Δ Base Up and 2Δ Base Left.

Measurement of addition in multifocals

When measuring the near addition of a bifocal or trifocal (Chapter 8), the distance prescription and centration should be measured in the same way as for a single vision lens. The power of the addition for any multifocal is the difference in spherical power between the distance and near portions of the lens, measured on the surface on which the addition is manufactured (BS 2738 Part 1, 1998). For example, the addition in a rear surface solid bifocal is the difference between distance and near back vertex powers, while the add in a front surface fused bifocal is the difference between distance and near front vertex powers. Therefore, in the latter example, the lenses should be placed front surface down on the focimeter to measure the near add, but rear surface down to measure the distance prescription. It is particularly important to measure the addition on the correct surface in lenses with high positive distance prescriptions.

With conventional invisible bifocals, the position of the near optical centre need not be measured, as its position cannot be specified.

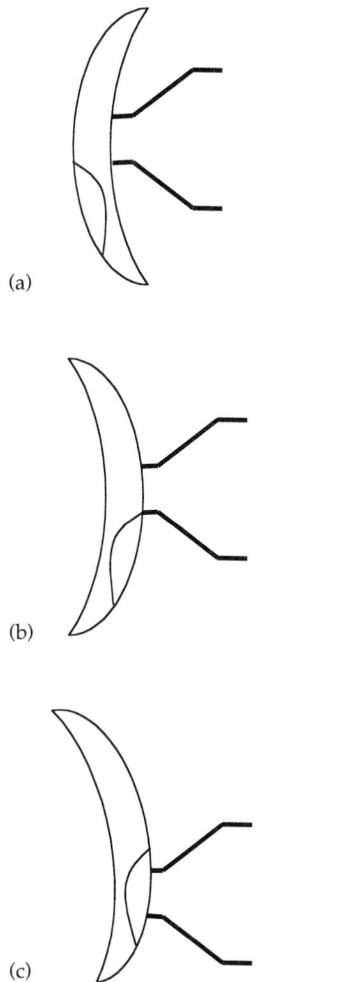

Figure 6.17. Measurement of addition for front surface multifocals. (a) BVP for distance; (b) FVP distance; (c) FVP near. Addition is FVP near minus FVP distance.

In some instances, particularly in negative prescriptions with large downcurve segments, there may be so much prism at near that the focimeter image cannot be seen. In this case a compensating prism can be inserted into the focimeter, or the near portion hand-neutralized.

Automatic focimeters

Although attempts were made to produce electromechanical automatic focimeters in the 1950s (see, for example Whitney, 1958), it was not until the development of microelectronics that such instruments became practical. The first commercial instrument was produced by Acuity Systems in the 1970s, and since then many others have been introduced.

The main feature of an automatic focimeter is that no visual focusing is required – the power is assessed completely electronically. A schematic diagram of an automatic focimeter is shown in Figure 6.18, and clearly the ray path is somewhat different from the conventional instrument, where parallel light exits the front surface of the unknown lens and enters the focimeter telescope. In the automatic instrument, parallel light from four light emitting diodes (A, B) enters the rear surface of the lens under test at L, the lens characteristics being assessed by how much, and in which direction, each of the four light beams is deviated at the sensor (S).

In order to centre a lens before making measurements, some form of indication is given as to the position of the optical centre,

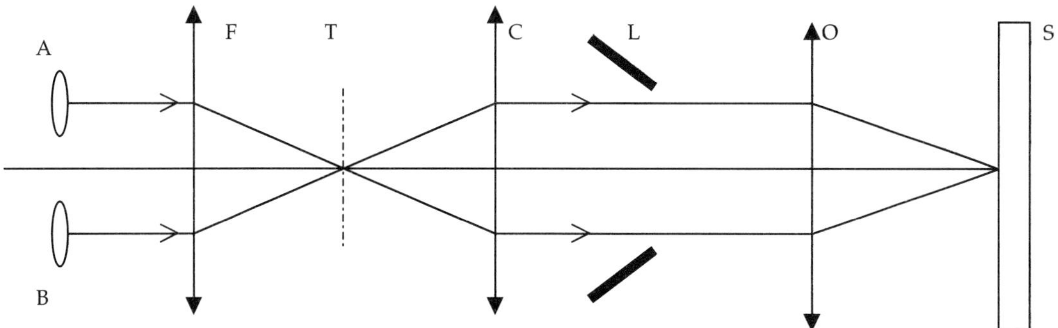

Figure 6.18. Schematic diagram of an automatic focimeter. A and B are two of the four LED light sources. Light from the target T is collimated by lens C. The lens to be measured is placed at L, and emergent light is imaged by lens O on to a sensor S. In some instruments, S may move along the optical axis of the instrument to find the best focus (Redrawn from a diagram provided by Nidek).

either by means of illuminated arrows, or by a simulation of the view seen in the telescope of a conventional focimeter, displayed on a computer screen. Instruments have variable rounding algorithms, so that readings can be displayed to the nearest 0.12 or 0.25 D. Some automated focimeters are capable of indicating to the nearest 0.01 D, although the instruments are not accurate to this value.

Accuracy of focimeters

No instrument is 100 per cent accurate, but this point does not always appear to have been grasped by users of focimeters. The problem of design in relation to the power of the collimating lens has already been discussed in this chapter, and some of the other points to be considered are discussed below.

Calibration wavelength

There are two wavelengths commonly used for focimeter calibration: 587.56 nm (helium 'd' line) and 546.07 nm (mercury 'e' line), as laid down in BS EN ISO 7944 (1998). Unfortunately, instruments do not normally state at which wavelength they were calibrated. The effect of using a different wavelength can be shown by an example. The refractive index of white ophthalmic crown glass is 1.523 for the 'd' line and 1.525 for the 'e' line. A –20.00 DS lens manufactured relative to the 'd' line would measure as –19.92 DS on a focimeter calibrated for the 'e' line.

Sagittal height error

The focimeter lens rest or 'nosepiece' does not quite give a fixed lens vertex position at the second principle focus of the collimating lens as indicated in the theory. Because the lens rest is an annular support for the lens there must be a finite diameter and, as shown in Figure 6.19, this can cause a displacement of the rear lens surface from the correct position in the case of steeply curved lens surfaces. This is mostly a problem in the case of contact lenses, and thus most focimeters use a special type of lens holder for this type of lens. It might be considered a solution to make the aperture of the lens support very small.

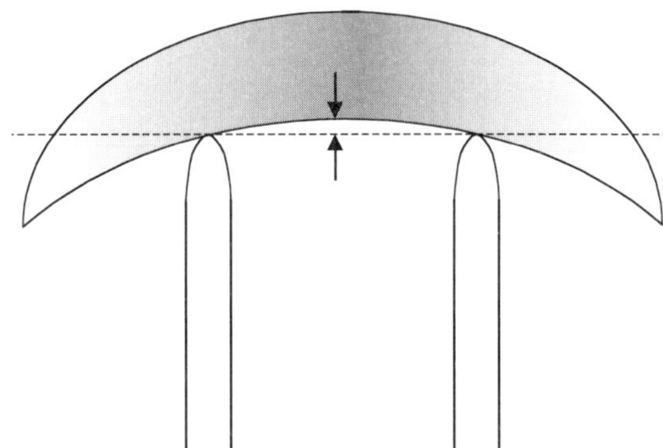

Figure 6.19. Sagittal height error for focimeter lens support.

Unfortunately this will increase the depth of focus of the instrument, giving a range of power readings where a sharp focus can be found. Many instruments use an aperture diameter of about 10 mm, with a smaller diameter being used for the measurement of contact lenses in order to reduce the sagittal height error. Conventional optical focimeters will also give a sharper image when measuring the near power of a progressive lens if a smaller focimeter aperture is used, as these lenses are very aspheric at near with a limited stable power.

Spherical aberration

Increasing the aperture diameter of the lens support will give a reduced depth of focus and make the lens power easier to find, but it will also sharply worsen the sagittal height error problem, and also make the spherical aberration of the lens being measured become more apparent.

Automatic focimeters

Although most automatic focimeters will indicate to 0.01 D, it should be emphasized that they are not accurate to this level. Most instruments have a best claimed accuracy (depending on the lens power) in the order of ±0.04 D.

A particular feature of automatic focimeters is that they typically use red solid state lasers as light sources. As the refractive index of normal lens materials is different at red wavelengths to the value at the 'd' or 'e' line, the instrument measures the 'wrong' power. However, the correct power is calculated and displayed by knowing the dispersion of normal lens materials and applying a correction factor. Early instruments assumed an Abbe value of 58 for this calculation, so that errors can occur on high refractive index materials with low constringence. More recent instruments can be set to any required Abbe number. This problem does not arise with visually focusing instruments, which utilize a filter to provide light of the correct wavelength.

Presentation of focimeter results

Prescription orders should conform to BS 2738-3 (1991). Most of this is common sense, but in outline is as follows:

- Give lens powers to two decimal places, with + or – sign as appropriate.
- Do not use a degree sign for the cyl axis, as this can be confused with a zero.
- The right eye is designated 'R', and information for this eye should be given first. The left eye is designated 'L', and information common to both eyes is designated 'BE'.
- Horizontal centration or monocular centrations should be stated. If vertical centrations are not stated, they are assumed to lie on the horizontal centre line (Chapter 4). Locations of segment top position and geometric inset for multifocals (Chapter 8) should also be given where relevant.
- An order is complete only when it includes the name and address of the patient, the name, address and signature of the prescriber, and the date.

Tolerances on glazed spectacles

The focimeter is often used to check the accuracy of a prescription before dispensing the spectacles to a patient. The prescription should be accurate according to BS 2738 Part 1 (1998), which specifies the tolerances that apply to the nominal values on the prescription order. Table 6.1 shows the tolerances on back vertex power for single vision lenses and the distance portion of multifocals. Tolerances on progressive power lenses are slightly more lenient. To use the table, consider the prescription in cross-cylinder form and consider the power of the meridian with highest absolute power. For example, in the prescription +2.00 DS/ –6.00 DC × 180, the meridian with highest absolute power is –4.00 DC × 180. Now by examining the relevant row in Table 6.1, the tolerance on each meridian is given by A, and the tolerance on the cylinder, or the difference between the two powers, is given by B. Tolerances on cyl axes and the additions for multifocal or progressive lenses are shown in Tables 6.2 and 6.3 respectively. Tolerances on centration and prismatic power are discussed in Chapter 4. If a pair of spectacles do not conform to these tolerances in any respect, then the work should be rejected.

Focimeter standards

An International Standard (BS EN ISO 8598, 1998) has been produced for the manufacturing accuracy of focimeters, covering both visually focusing and automated designs. According to this standard, a focimeter

Table 6.1 Tolerances on the back vertex power of single vision and multifocal glazed lenses as applied to the nominal values on the prescription order. All values are in D. (Taken from BS 2738–1, 1998)

Power of meridian with highest absolute power	*Tolerance on the power of each meridian, A*	*Tolerance on the cylindrical power, B*			
		≥ 0.00 and ≤ 0.75	*> 0.75 and ≤ 4.00*	*> 4.00 and ≥ 6.00*	*> 6.00*
≥ 0.00 and ≤ 3.00	±0.12	±0.09	±0.12	±0.18	±0.25
> 3.00 and ≤ 6.00	±0.12	±0.12	±0.12	±0.18	±0.25
> 6.00 and ≤ 9.00	±0.12	±0.12	±0.18	±0.18	±0.25
> 9.00 and ≤ 12.00	±0.18	±0.12	±0.18	±0.25	±0.25
> 12.00 and ≤ 20.00	±0.25	±0.18	±0.25	±0.25	±0.25
> 20.00	±0.37	±0.25	±0.25	±0.37	±0.37

Table 6.2 Tolerances on the direction of the cylinder axis as applied to the nominal values on the prescription order. All values are in D. (Taken from BS 2738–1, 1998)

Cylinder power (D)	*Tolerance on the cylinder axis (°)*
≤ 0.50	±7
> 0.50 and ≤ 0.75	±5
> 0.75 and ≤ 1.50	±3
> 1.50	±2

Table 6.3 Tolerances on the addition power of multifocal and progressive power lenses, as applied to the nominal values on the prescription order. All values are in D. (Taken from BS 2738–1, 1998)

Value of the addition power	*Tolerance*
≤ 4.00	±0.12
> 4.00	±0.18

should be capable of measuring vertex powers up to at least ±20 D and prism up to at least 5Δ. The focimeter should meet the required accuracy standards for both the mercury 'e' line (546.07 nm) and the helium 'd' line (587.56 nm) reference wavelengths (BS EN ISO 7944, 1998). If not, then the wavelength used for calibration should be specified on the instrument.

The accuracy requirements are divided into those for continuously indicating instruments (those with an analogue scale) and those for digitally indicating instruments. The division is made because the majority of digital instruments cannot display the lens power to a finer increment than 0.125 D. Tables 6.4–6.7 are adapted from BS EN ISO 8598 (1998).

In order to test a focimeter to the required levels of accuracy a set of known power test lenses is required, and BS EN ISO 9342 (1998) gives the required tolerances for such a set. A set of 10 lenses is recommended for vertex power, with powers ranging from 5 to 25 D in 5 D steps in both plus and minus. The lens forms are chosen to be close to those commonly used in commercial spectacle lenses, so that spherical aberration values are similar. The tolerances given are extremely tight, thus in the case of the –10, –5 and +5

Table 6.4 Tolerances of measured vertex power for continuously indicating focimeters. All values are in dioptres (D). (From BS EN ISO 8598, 1998)

Measuring range of vertex power	*Tolerance*
> 0 to 5	±0.06
> 5 to 10	±0.09
> 10 to 15	±0.12
> 15 to 20	±0.18
> 20	±0.25

Table 6.5 Tolerances of measured prismatic power for continuously indicating focimeters. All values are in prism dioptres (Δ). (From BS EN ISO 8598, 1998)

Measuring range of prismatic power	*Tolerance*
> 0 to 5	0.1
> 5 to 10	0.2
> 10 to 15	0.3
> 15 to 20	0.4
> 20	0.5

Table 6.6 Permissible deviation of measured vertex power from the nominal value of the test lenses for digitally indicating focimeters. All values in dioptres (D). (From BS EN ISO 8598, 1998)

Measuring range of vertex power	*Deviation from nominal value of the test lens*	
	Increments of 0.25	*Increments of 0.25*
	0.25	*0.125*
> 0 to 5	0.0	0.0
> 5 to 10	0.0	±0.125
> 10 to 15	0.0	±0.125
> 15 to 20	±0.25	±0.125
> 20	±0.25	±0.25

Table 6.7 Permissible deviations of measured prismatic power readings from nominal value of the test lenses for digitally indicating focimeters. All values are in prism dioptres (Δ). (From BS EN ISO 8598, 1998)

Measuring range of prismatic power	*Deviation*	
	Increments of 0.25	*Increments of 0.125*
> 0 to 5	0.0	0.125
> 5 to 15	0.25	0.25
> 15 to 20	0.5	0.375
> 20	0.5	0.5

lenses, which cover the majority of prescription lenses, the lenses will have a tolerance of no more than ±0.01 D from the nominal. It is extremely difficult to measure lens powers to these tolerances, thus in the appendix to ISO 9342 a method is described of producing a set of lenses by strict parameter control. Thus if the refractive index of the lens material is accurately known, the thickness can be readily measured and controlled to a high standard, and the surface curves compared to known test plates by Newton ring methods, then the finished lens can be readily computed to a known power. Unfortunately this gives rise to a very expensive set of lenses.

An alternative method is to take a set of mass-produced lenses and have them accurately calibrated in a metrology laboratory. For example, the National Physical Laboratory in the United Kingdom will calibrate the vertex powers of lenses and issue a certificate. For a set of test lenses used by the authors, the certificate states that the lenses are calibrated to 'an accuracy of ±0.02 D at a confidence level of 99%'.

Besides the vertex power set of test lenses, BS EN ISO 9342 (1998) specifies a set of test plano prisms, and a special plano cylinder with an accurately machined flat base parallel to the cylinder axis, used for testing the accuracy of the frame table and marking device.

Summary

In this chapter, hand neutralization and the focimeter have been discussed as methods for measuring parameters of spectacle lenses. In addition to measuring vertex power, the optical centre, cylinder axes, prism and near vision addition can be determined using either method.

Formulae

Formula	*Name*	*Equation number*
$f^2 = -x.x'$	Newton's relationship	6.01
$x = \frac{1000}{F^2}$	Focimeter target travel	6.02

Exercises

Questions

1. A sphero-cylindrical lens is hand neutralized. Meridian A is neutralized by a −2.00 D lens and meridian B is neutralized by a −4.00 D lens. Using a protractor, meridian 'B' is found to be at an axis of 120. What is the power of the lens in sphero-cylindrical form?
2. A sphero-cylindrical lens is rotated in plan view and scissors distortion is observed. Meridian A rotates 'with' the lens rotation and meridian B rotates 'against' the lens rotation. The transverse movements for meridians A and B are both 'with' movements. Which meridian corresponds to the negative cyl axis?
3. A tangent scale is viewed through a prism of power 2Δ held at a distance of 2 m from the scale. How far will the image of the scale be deviated by viewing it through the prism?
4. A focimeter has a standard lens of power +35 DS.
   a. What is the movement in mm for each 1.00 D reading on the power scale?
   b. What is (theoretically) the maximum positive power that this focimeter can read?
   c. Given that the graticule can be marked in steps equivalent to 1 mm of target travel, what are the graduations in terms of lens power?
5. A focimeter has a standard lens power of +15 DS.
   a. What is the movement in mm for each 1.00 D reading on the power scale?
   b. What is (theoretically) the maximum positive power that this focimeter can read?
   c. Given that the graticule can be marked in steps equivalent to 1 mm of target travel, what are the graduations in terms of lens power?
6. A focimeter has a standard lens power of +25 DS.
   a. What is the movement in mm for each 1.00 D reading on the power scale?
   b. The instrument will read between powers of +20.00 DS and −24.00 DS. What is the total travel of the target in mm between these powers?

c. The focimeter is used to measure the back vertex powers of a lens of power +5.00 DS/−2.50 DC × 90. The focimeter is adjusted to bring the +5.00 D meridian into focus. Draw the type of image you would expect to observe. To bring the other meridian into focus, how far will the target have to travel?

7. Given your results from Questions 3–5, what standard lens would make the best focimeter? Why?
8. The power of a plano-convex lens of refractive index 1.5 is measured on a focimeter. When the lens is placed rear surface down on the focimeter, the power reading is +15 D. When the lens is placed front surface down, the power reading is +14 D. What is the centre thickness of the lens?
9. The back vertex power of a crown glass lens measured on a focimeter calibrated according to the mercury 'e' line is +15.00 D. What is the power of the lens if a focimeter is used that is calibrated according to the helium 'd' line?
10. What tolerance would you accept on a glazed prescription of +7.00 DS/+5.00 DC × 90 Add +3.00 D?

Answers

1. +4.00 DS/−2.00 DC × 30
2. Meridian A
3. 4 cm
4. a) 0.82 mm/D; b) +35 DS; c) 1.225 D
5. a) 4.44 mm/D; b) +15 DS; c) 0.225 D
6. a) 1.6 mm/D; b) 70.4 mm; c) 4 mm
8. 7.14 mm
9. +14.94 D
10. On +12.00 D meridian, ±0.18 D; on +7.00 D meridian, ±0.18 D; on 5.00 DC cylindrical power, ±0.25 D. Axis ±2°, addition power ±0.12 D.

7

Lens aberrations, best form and aspheric lenses

Lens aberrations

All lenses are affected by aberrations, reducing image quality from that theoretically possible. There are now a number of different ways of assessing image quality and lens aberrations, but the traditional approach of Seidel is perhaps the most familiar in spectacle lenses.

The Seidel aberrations are divided into two groups, *axial* and *transverse* (or oblique), depending on whether the object is positioned on or off the lens axis. The aberrations can also be classified as monochromatic or polychromatic, depending on the wavelengths of light being considered.

Axial aberrations

Spherical

Spherical aberration is an aberration of large aperture systems, where different zones of the lens have different focal lengths. In Figure 7.1, the focal length of rays entering close to the axis is longer than the focal length for peripheral rays. Although the aperture of spectacle lenses is often large in relation to their focal lengths, only a small area is viewed by the eye at any one time. Spherical aberration is therefore not normally considered in the design of spectacle lenses.

Chromatic

Axial chromatic aberration is depicted in Figure 7.2 and was discussed in Chapter 5. In essence, the aberration arises because blue light is refracted more than red light by a material of any given refractive index (Chapter 1). As the human eye exhibits chromatic aberration in the order of 0.75 D, this aberration is not normally noticed with current spectacle lens materials.

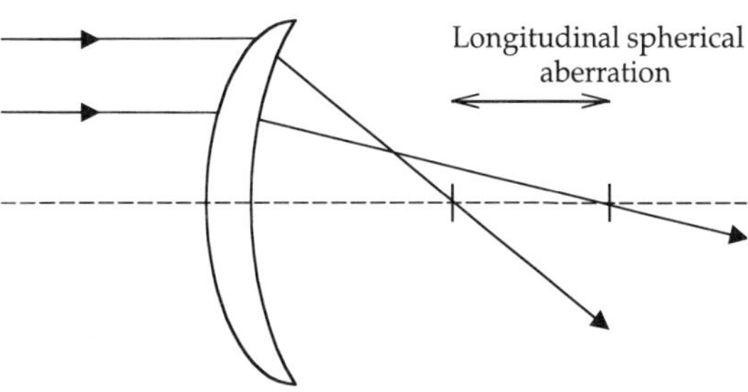

Figure 7.1. Axial, or longitudinal, spherical aberration in a spectacle lens. The paraxial rays have a longer focal length than the more peripheral rays.

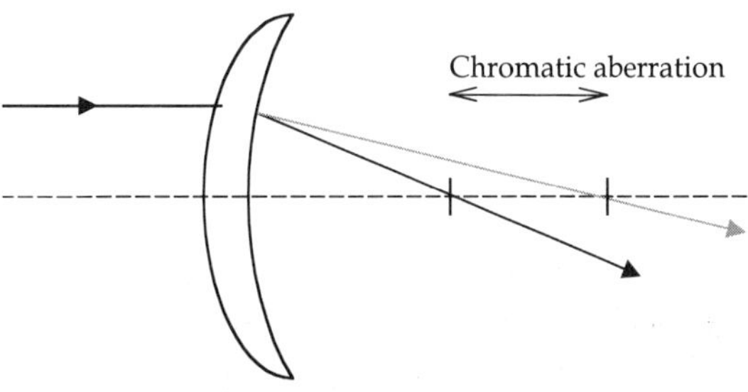

Figure 7.2. Axial chromatic aberration in a spectacle lens. The lens material has a higher refractive index for short wavelengths than for longer wavelengths of light.

Oblique aberrations

Coma

Coma is so called because of the appearance of the image, which is like a bright comet with a flared tail (Figure 7.3). As with spherical aberration, this is a problem in larger aperture optical systems, but is not considered in spectacle lens design.

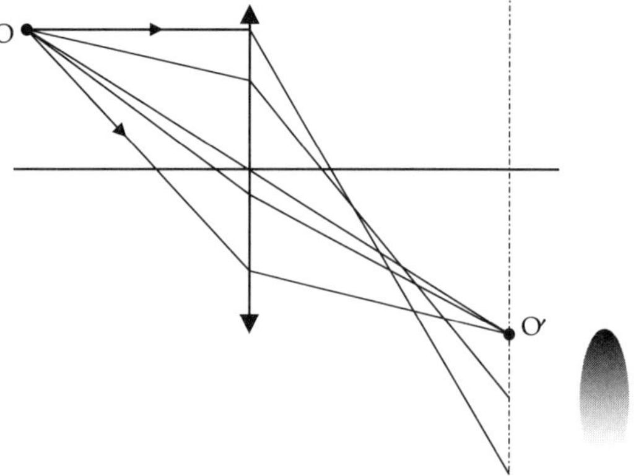

Figure 7.3. Coma, or oblique spherical aberration, in a spectacle lens. The off-axis point object forms an image with comatous flare.

Transverse chromatic aberration

Transverse chromatic aberration can be a problem in lens powers over 5.00 D where materials of low (less than 45) Abbe number are used (Chapter 5). This can result in blurred vision off-axis, as well as colour fringing on high contrast borders. Varying the lens form can have a small effect on this aberration.

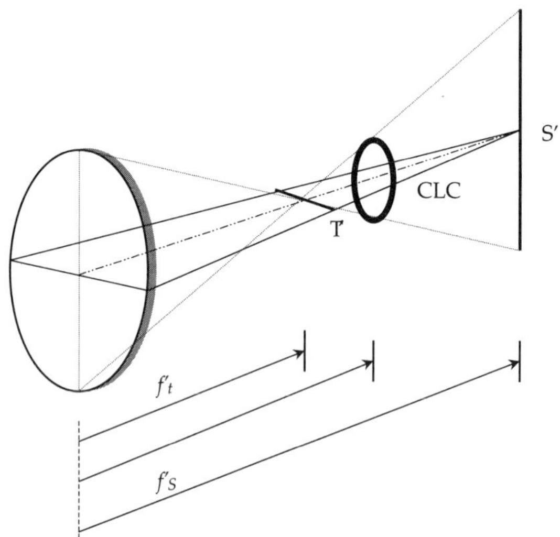

Figure 7.4. Oblique astigmatism in a spectacle lens. View of an oblique pencil of light. Note that the whole lens is not represented. Rays of light entering the lens obliquely from a point object form two line foci, the tangential (T′) and sagittal (S′) images, with focal lengths f'_t and f'_s respectively.

Oblique astigmatism

Oblique astigmatism is due solely to obliquely incident light, and has historically been one of the major concerns of spectacle lens designers. In Figure 7.4, light is obliquely incident on a lens from a distant object. Rays in the plane of the paper (entering the lens at the top and bottom) form a line image, the *tangential* (T′), so called because it is formed tangential to the rim of the lens. Rays in a perpendicular section to the plane of the paper (entering on the left and right sides of the lens) form the *sagittal* image (S′), aligned to a sagittal section of the lens. In between these two line images is the *circle of least confusion*. For a single surface, the positions of the foci can be determined by *Young's construction*. In Figure 7.5, an object off the axis at O is incident at point P of a refracting surface, where the centre of curvature is at C. A line through O and C will, where it cuts the refracted ray, give the position of the sagittal focus, S′. In Figure 7.6, the additional construction lines for the tangential focus are shown. A perpendicular is drawn from C to the incident ray, produced if necessary, at point A, and a second perpendicular is drawn from C to the refracted ray, at point B. A third perpendicular is drawn from C to a line through A and B, to produce point D. A line through O and D will then give the position of the tangential image T′ where it cuts the refracted ray. For a distant object, construction lines parallel to the chief ray incident at P would be drawn through C and D.

Although it would be theoretically possible to find the positions of the foci in a lens using Young's construction, in practice this is difficult to achieve with any degree of accuracy, so that computer ray tracing is now universally used. Figure 7.7 illustrates the computing

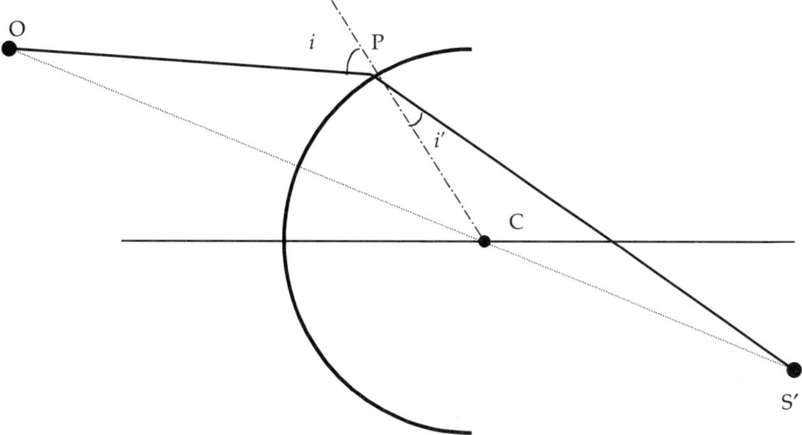

Figure 7.5. Young's construction showing the position of the sagittal image S′, when the point object is at O and the centre of curvature of the single lens surface is at C.

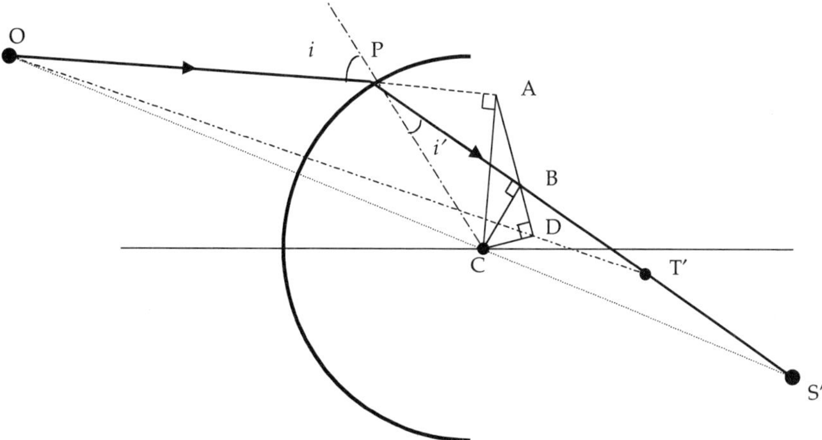

Figure 7.6. Young's construction showing the position of the tangential image T′, when the point object is at O, the centre of curvature of the single lens surface is at C and the sagittal image is positioned at S′.

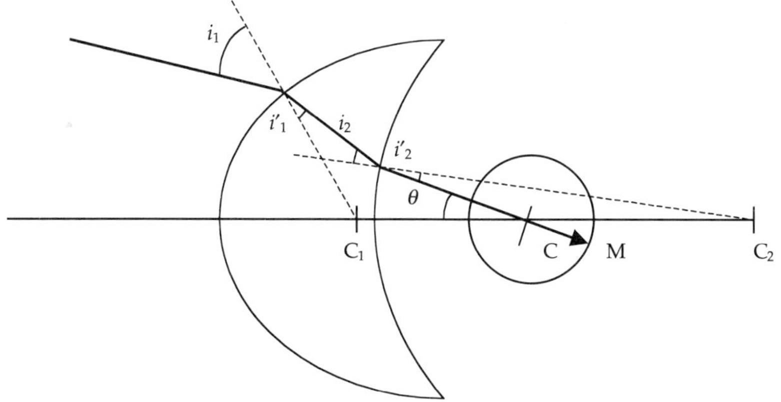

Figure 7.7. Ray tracing method for the determination of sagittal and tangential image positions when an oblique point object is viewed through a lens.

method. A ray is first traced backwards through the system at a given angle θ to the lens axis, starting from the centre of rotation of the eye (CR). At each surface, the angles of incidence (i) and refraction (i') are calculated. The sagittal image position for each surface can then be found from:

$$\frac{n'}{s'} - \frac{n}{s} = \frac{n' \cos i' - n \cos i}{r} \qquad \textit{Equation 7.01}$$

and the tangential from:

$$\frac{n' \cos^2 i'}{t'} - \frac{n \cos^2 i}{t} = \frac{n' \cos i' - n \cos i}{r} \qquad \textit{Equation 7.02}$$

where s is the sagittal object distance, s' is the distance of the sagittal image from the lens surface, t is the tangential object distance, t' is the distance of the tangential image from the lens surface, and r is the radius of curvature of the lens surface.

These equations are applied to each surface in turn, with due allowance being made for lens thickness. The sagittal (S'_v) and tangential image vergences (T'_v) are conventionally calculated not from the rear surface of the lens, but from the locus of the vertex distance from the centre of rotation, known as the *vertex sphere* (see Figure 7.9).

Oblique astigmatism is an important consideration in the design of spectacle lenses. Excess amounts of oblique astigmatism are seen by the observer as blur through the edges of their spectacle lenses, as would

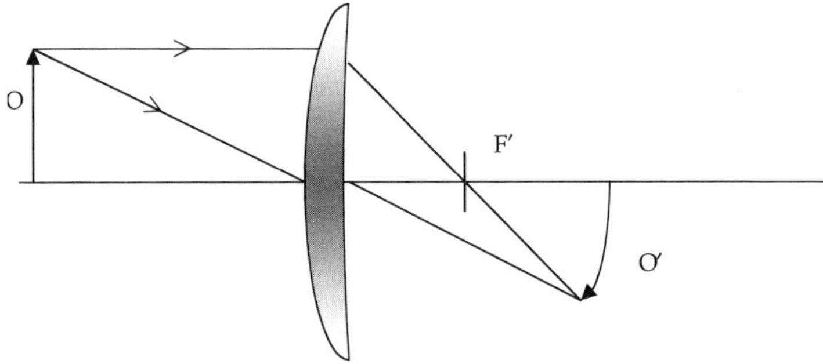

Figure 7.8. Curvature of a spectacle lens demonstrated with an extended object. The flat object is imaged in a curved plane.

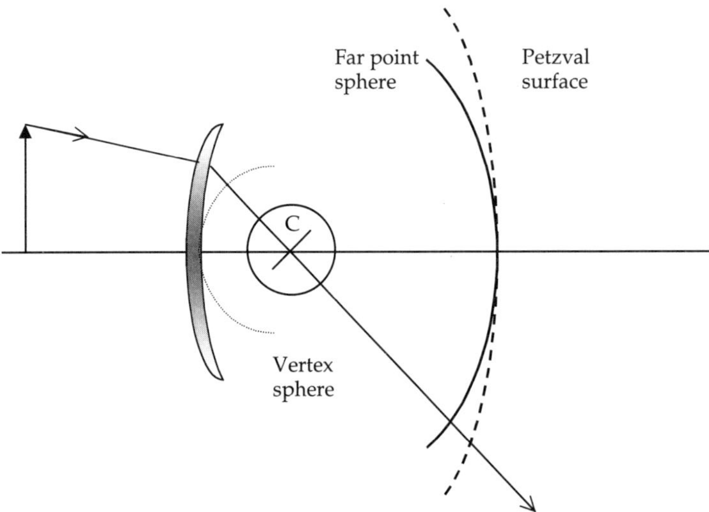

Figure 7.9. Curved image planes. The far point sphere is the image plane of the eye for macular vision. The Petzval surface is the curved image plane for the lens. The vertex sphere is the locus of points equidistant from the centre of rotation of the eye and is equivalent to the paraxial vertex distance.

be seen with an uncorrected cylindrical refractive error. The blur is particularly noticeable when viewing high contrast edges. Alleviation of the effects of oblique astigmatism in spectacle lenses is discussed later in this chapter.

Curvature of field

If a lens suffers from field curvature, then the image of a flat object will be produced in a curved plane (Figure 7.8). This aberration is a problem in camera lenses, where the image plane is flat film, but is a positive advantage in spectacle lenses where the image plane for macular vision is the curved *far point sphere.* In the absence of oblique astigmatism, the curved image plane is known as the *Petzval surface* (Figure 7.9), and would ideally coincide with the far point sphere. Unfortunately this only happens in one unique case for a given lens power, refractive index and centre of rotation distance. In all other cases there is a power error, and the image formed on the Petzval surface is not coincident with the far point sphere. To the observer, there is blur through the edges of their spectacle lenses as if there were an uncorrected spherical refractive error. Curvature of field, or mean oblique error, is therefore a consideration in spectacle lens design.

Distortion

An image which is affected by distortion is perfectly sharp, is positioned in the correct plane, but is not the correct shape. Distortion can be considered as variable magnification across the lens aperture, and is a significant problem in higher power spectacle lenses.

In Figure 7.10, an eye has rotated through an angle u to view the extremity of an object. The effective angle of rotation is u', and for a distortion free lens the value of ($\tan u'/\tan u$) should be a constant for all angles of gaze. If the ratio is less than unity, then barrel distor-

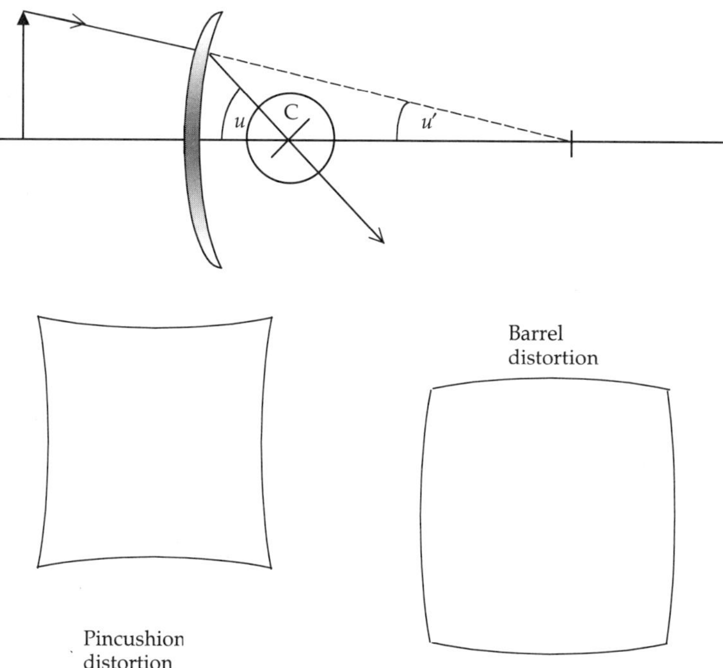

Figure 7.10. Distortion in a spectacle lens. The upper part of the figure shows an eye that has rotated through angle u to view a peripheral ray of ray entering the lens. The effective angle of gaze is u'. The lower part of the figure shows the effects of distortion. If the ratio of $\tan u'/\tan u$ is greater than unity for the peripheral parts of the lens, as is the case with positive lenses, then pincushion distortion results. If the ratio is less than unity, as with negative lenses, then barrel distortion results.

tion is demonstrated, typically associated with negative lenses. Positive lenses tend to show pincushion distortion, where the ratio of tan u'/tan u is greater than unity.

Thus a myope will tend to see the walls bulging outwards, the ceiling upwards, and the floor downwards, when looking down a corridor wearing lenses with significant barrel distortion. A hypermetrope will experience the opposite effect.

Controlling aberrations in spectacle lenses

From the above discussion it will be seen that the significant aberrations for a spectacle lens are transverse chromatic aberration, oblique astigmatism, curvature and distortion. As far as chromatic aberration is concerned, the only effective means of control is by choice of a suitable lens material with a high enough Abbe number (Chapter 5). Unfortunately there is no simple way of deciding what is the optimum value for a given individual. Quite simply, some lens wearers are bothered by transverse chromatic aberration, but many are not.

Oblique astigmatism is a major cause of poor visual acuity when objects are viewed through the edge of a lens. Fortunately this aberration is very sensitive to changes in lens form, and can be reduced to zero in most prescriptions by the use of a suitable base curve. Although trigonometric ray tracing as described in the previous section gives the most accurate estimation of oblique astigmatism, thin lens and small angle approximations give a very good prediction of the best lens form. In Figure 7.11 a graph known as *Tscherning's ellipse* is shown. This is the solution of a quadratic equation for zero oblique astigmatism, assuming:

- The lens is thin
- A small oblique angle of gaze, such that 'third order' approximations can be made
- A specific refractive index for the lens
- A specific centre of rotation distance (z)
- A specific fixation distance, in this case infinity.

Thus in the range of powers with a real solution for the quadratic, there are two forms for zero oblique astigmatism for any given back vertex power. The steep form (Wollaston), with a highly powered rear surface (F_2), is shown by the lower portion of the curve. The shallower form (Ostwalt) is shown by the upper portion. In fact, even the shallow forms are much steeper in form than curves commonly used today for spectacle lenses. One reason for this is that single vision lenses are commonly used for a wide variety of fixation distances and, as shown in Figure

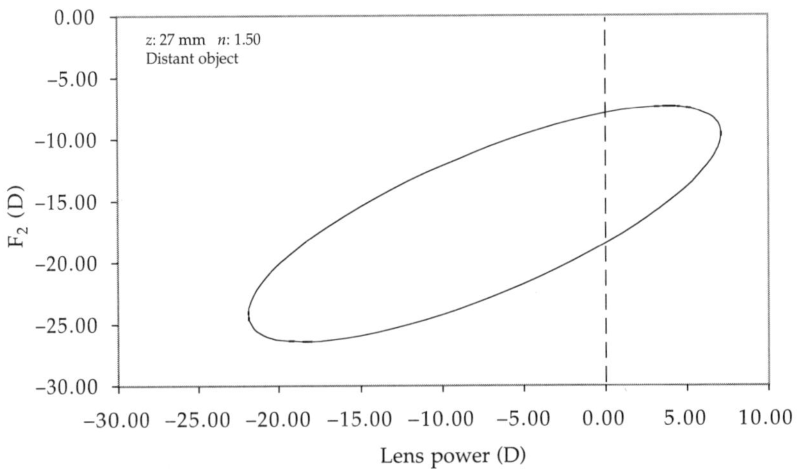

Figure 7.11. Tscherning's ellipse for a distant object viewed through a lens of refractive index (n) 1.50 by an eye whose centre of rotation (z) is 27 mm from the lens. The ellipse gives the rear surface power(s) (F_2) that a lens of any given back vertex power (F'_v) should have in order to eliminate oblique astigmatism.

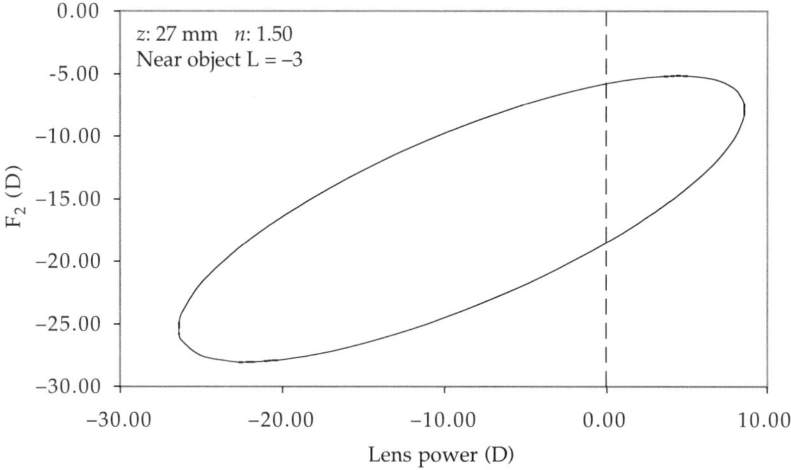

Figure 7.12. Tscherning's ellipse for the same conditions as Figure 7.11, except that the object viewed is at 33 cm from the lens. Note that although the lens properties remain constant, the ideal rear surface curves change with this change in viewing distance.

7.12, changing the fixation distance to a near object produces a significant change in lens form. Some examples of the third order lens forms for different prescriptions are shown in Table 7.1. Note that the near vision forms for a fixation distance of one-third of a metre (incident vergence $L = -3$) require flatter forms of lens than for distance fixation. Thus a general purpose lens series must be a compromise between the requirements of distance and near vision.

If the refractive index changes, then this can also require a change in lens form to maintain zero oblique astigmatism. Table 7.2 illustrates this by comparing lenses in both normal index (1.50) and high index (1.70) materials. In each case the reading of a lens measure calibrated for $n = 1.523$ is also given for the front surface, to illustrate the physical change in lens form required when changing refractive index. Note that in the case of the +5.00 lens the front curve is physically flatter with the high refractive index, but the

Table 7.1 Solutions of Tscherning's ellipse for lenses of different back vertex power, and for two fixation distances (distance, and 33 cm). The lenses are made of 1.5 index material, with a centre of rotation distance (z) of 27 mm. To eliminate oblique astigmatism, the rear surface of the lens should have a rear surface power (F_2) of one of the solutions given

Third–order lens forms – zero oblique astigmatism

Lens power	F_2 *(shallow)*	F_2 *(steep)*
	Distance vision (L = 0)	
–10.00	–12.18	–24.28
–6.00	–10.11	–22.35
–2.00	–8.52	–19.93
+2.00	–7.54	–16.92
+5.00	–7.52	–13.94
+7.00	–8.88	–10.58
	Near vision (L = –3)	
–10.00	–9.78	–24.53
–6.00	–7.87	–22.45
–2.00	–6.36	–19.95
+2.00	–5.38	–16.94
+5.00	–5.17	–14.14
+7.00	–5.58	–11.73

Table 7.2 Variations in lens form required for lenses free of oblique astigmatism when lens power and refractive index are varied. The observer is viewing a distant target and the centre of rotation distance (z) is a constant 27 mm

Normal and high index lenses

Lens power	*n*	F_2	F_1	F_1*(1.523)*
+5.00	1.50	–7.52	+12.52	+13.10
+5.00	1.70	–12.02	+17.02	+12.72
–5.00	1.50	–9.66	+4.66	+4.87
–5.00	1.70	–13.15	+8.15	+6.09

Third–order lens forms free from oblique astigmatism.

opposite is true with the –5.00 lens. Thus care must be taken when changing refractive index of lens materials.

Table 7.2 also illustrates the point that even the flatter of the two possible astigmatism free forms is still steeply curved. When spectacle frames are small with small lens sizes this is not a major concern, as the cosmetic appearance is not such a problem with steep lens forms. However, for over 25 years at the latter end of the twentieth century fashionable spectacle frames used large lens sizes, which naturally had an influence on lens form. First of all steep lens forms in large diameters make the lens look unattractive, and secondly high power lenses are restricted in maximum diameter in such forms (Chapter 2).

There are other philosophies for lens design besides attaining zero oblique astigmatism. Two other design criteria in particular have been promoted. The first of these is zero mean power error. Oblique astigmatism is allowed, but the circle of least confusion is placed on the far point sphere. Such lenses are sometimes called Percival designs after the ophthalmologist who promoted the concept. A second approach is to have minimum tangential error, so that the tangential focus is placed on the far point sphere, at the expense of the sagittal image focus.

These different philosophies are illustrated in Table 7.3, where a +5.00 D lens is shown in different forms corresponding to the different design concepts. Note that the Percival form of lens is the flattest (lowest power on the rear surface), while the steeper forms have reduced distortion. With spherical surface curves, distortion can only be minimized in this lens. Note that the steeper of the two astigmatism-free lenses with a rear surface power of –12.12 D is a very good all round compromise optically, but it would be poor cosmetically and only capable of manufacture in very small diameters due to the steep surface powers. Table 7.3 also illustrates the fact that Tscherning's ellipse only gives an approximate indication of the exact lens form calculated by ray tracing. The table of designs corresponding to different philosophies for a –5.00 DS lens is shown in Table 7.4.

Table 7.3 The effect of different lens forms on optical aberrations of a +5.00 DS lens of 1.5 index material, viewed with an eye with a centre of rotation distance (z) of 27 mm and an angle of rotation from the optical axis of 35°

F_2	*Ast (D)*	*MOP (D)*	*DIST (%)*	S'_v	T'_v	*Lens type*
–3.60	0.39	5.00	7.73	4.81	5.20	Percival
–4.25	0.25	4.88	7.25	4.75	5.00	Minimum tangential error
–5.94	0.00	4.64	6.19	4.64	4.64	Zero astigmatism flat form
–12.12	0.00	4.59	4.13	4.59	4.59	Zero astigmatism steep form
–14.00	0.24	4.80	4.00	4.68	4.92	Minimum distortion

F_2, rear surface power required to fulfil the design criteria; AST, oblique astigmatism in dioptres; MOP, mean oblique power of the lens (the deviation of this value from +5.00 D indicates the curvature error); DIST, amount of distortion in the lens (%); S'_v, sagittal power; T'_v, tangential power.

Table 7.4 The effect of different lens forms on optical aberrations of a –5.00 DS lens of 1.5 index material, viewed with an eye with a centre of rotation distance (z) of 27 mm and an angle of rotation from the optical axis of 35°

F_2	*Ast (D)*	*MOP (D)*	*DIST (%)*	S'_v	T'_v	*Lens type*
–7.53	–0.26	–5.00	–8.65	–4.87	–5.13	Percival
–7.92	–0.17	–4.92	–8.29	–4.83	–5.00	Zero tangential error
–8.80	0.00	–4.76	–7.55	–4.76	–4.76	Zero astigmatism (shallow)
–21.50	0.00	–4.78	–2.97	–4.78	–4.78	Zero astigmatism (steep)
–23.50	–0.30	–5.08	–2.90	–4.93	–5.24	Minimum distortion

F_2, rear surface power required to fulfil the design criteria; AST, oblique astigmatism in dioptres; MOP, mean oblique power of the lens (the deviation of this value from +5.00 D indicates the curvature error); DIST, amount of distortion in the lens (%); S'_v, sagittal power; T'_v, tangential power. Angle of eye rotation 35°.

A lens that is designed to have some control of aberration is sometimes known as *best form*. As this description is often used somewhat indiscriminately, it is worth considering the British Standard definition (BS 3521, Part 1, 1991):

> *Best form lens: a lens whose curvatures are computed to eliminate or minimize a stated image defect or defects under defined conditions.*

Thus a best form lens may only attempt to reduce a single aberration for a given fixation distance. It is not guaranteed to be the best optical (or cosmetic) solution for a given prescription. In the USA, best form lenses are known as *corrected curve lenses*.

Aspheric lenses

Introduction

Aspheric lenses are lenses where at least one of the surfaces is made aspherical. Literally speaking, an aspherical surface could be any surface that is non-spherical in form, so could include cylindrical or toroidal surfaces. Equally, progressive power lens surfaces are aspherical in nature, but vary in their characteristics in different parts of the lens. We are therefore going to define the lenses discussed in this chapter as having *one surface that is of rotationally symmetrical aspherical form*. These lens forms were originally used exclusively for single vision lenses, but more recently bifocal lens forms have also become available.

However, first of all, why use these lens forms at all? Aspherical surfaces are more expensive to manufacture than spherical, and they are difficult to check accurately. The advantages were originally optical, have also become cosmetic, and there are some definite commercial benefits as well.

Development of aspheric lenses

The use of such surfaces had been suggested by Descartes in the seventeenth century, as a generalized approach to overcoming problems in optical systems, not necessarily spectacles. However, it was at the beginning of the twentieth century that interest was first shown in using this type of technology for spectacle lenses.

The Swedish ophthalmologist Alvar Gullstrand suggested to Moritz von Rohr of the Carl Zeiss company in Jena, Germany, that the use of an aspherical surface would improve the optical performance of high power spectacle lenses. It had already been shown by Airy in 1827, Tscherning in 1904 (cited by Bennett, 1965) and others that a spherical surface lens could not be made free from oblique astigmatism where the power was more than about +7.00 D. This is apparent from the Tscherning's ellipse, as shown in Figures 7.11 and 7.12. Von Rohr produced a UK patent in 1909 for both high positive and high negative power lenses. Interestingly, the patent also suggested the use of high refractive index glass. The patent advocated the use of a lens for high plus powers with a *rear* aspheric surface, the opposite of present day practice. No information was given on the geometry of the aspheric curve, but it is possible to show that the curve was closely equivalent to a conic section of revolution (Fowler, 1984).

The lens design of von Rohr would undoubtedly have been very expensive to produce by the conventional glass techniques of lapping, smoothing and polishing, so it was not until plastic materials came into common use that the use of aspheric surface lenses became widespread. This was because one glass aspherical mould could mould many CR39 lenses. At the same time, developments were taking place in the geometry of lens surfaces which also increased the use of aspheric lenses. For example, Welsh (1978) proposed a design of lens where the aspheric surface was composed of a series of intersecting spherical curves of similar radius.

Geometry of aspheric surfaces

The most straightforward aspheric surface is the conic section, shown in Figure 7.13. The terminology used by Baker (1943) is particularly convenient for optical computation of this type of surface. With the origin of an x, y coordinate system at the vertex of a surface (Figure 7.13), the curve is defined as:

$$y^2 = 2r_0x - px^2 \qquad \textit{Equation 7.03}$$

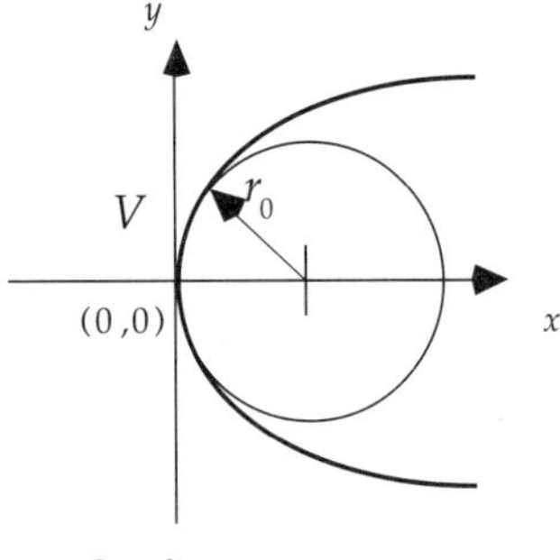

Figure 7.13. The terminology of a conic section. The apex or vertex (V) of the lens is at (0, 0) on a cartesian co-ordinate system, where y represents vertical displacement from the apex, and x represents horizontal displacement. The value r_0 is the radius of curvature of the sphere at the vertex of the lens. Note that the radius of curvature as y increases is not the same as that at r_0. The value p describes how the peripheral curvature compares to the vertex radius of curvature.

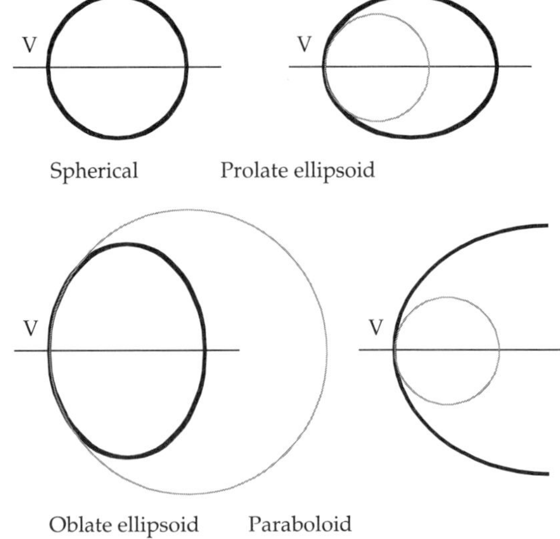

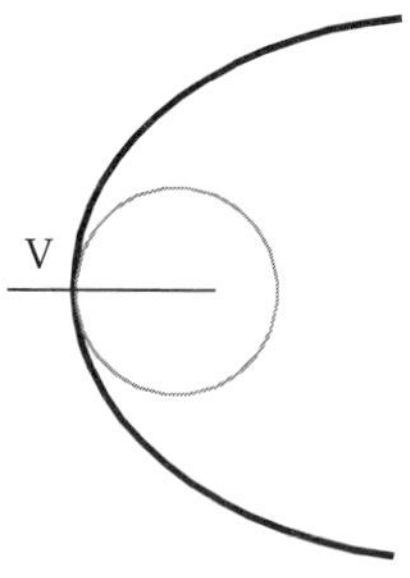

Figure 7.14. Diagrammatic representation of conic surfaces of different value of p (solid lines). The dotted lines show the spherical curvature of the vertex of the section (r_0). Note that the hyperboloid, paraboloid and prolate ellipsoid (p values <1) have a shallower peripheral curvature than the vertex sphere. The oblate ellipsoid (p >1) has a steeper peripheral curvature than at its vertex.

where r_0 is the paraxial radius of curvature, and p is the conic coefficient of the surface. The relationship of conic coefficients to various types of conic surface is given below:

$p < 0$ Hyperboloid
$p = 0$ Paraboloid
$1 > p > 0$ Prolate ellipsoid
$p = 1$ Spherical
$p > 1$ Oblate ellipsoid

The types of curve yielded by these various forms are shown in Figure 7.14. The peripheral flattening of the lens is the amount by which a curve departs from the spherical, as shown by the dotted lines in Figure 7.14, towards the edge of the lens. Note that in terms of peripheral flattening, the order is in relation to the value of p. Thus a hyperboloid will have the flattest aspheric form for a given value of r_0. It is sometimes more convenient to use the form of equation solved for x:

$$x = \frac{\frac{y^2}{r_0}}{1 + \sqrt{1 - p\left(\frac{y^2}{r_0^2}\right)}} \qquad \textit{Equation 7.04}$$

Aspheric surfaces are useful in ophthalmic optics, as they neutralize the oblique astigmatism caused by off-axis viewing by means of the astigmatism inherent in the surface. Thus any point apart from the optical centre will have surface astigmatism. This can be calculated for the tangential and sagittal meridians of the surface in terms of the localized radius in each meridian. The sagittal radius (r_s) is given by:

$$r_s = [r_0^2 + (1 - p)y^2]^{1/2} \qquad \textit{Equation 7.05}$$

and from this the tangential radius (r_t) is given by:

$$r_t = \frac{r_s^3}{r_0^2} \qquad \textit{Equation 7.06}$$

Table 7.5 Aberration values for +14.00 lens made with various front surface conic asphericities

Lens aberrations	
$F'v$	14.00
F_2	−2.00
t (mm)	10.00
n	1.50
z (mm)	27.00
Angle (°)	35.00
p_2	1.00

Front surface asphericity (p1)	*Oblique astigmatism*	*Mean oblique power (D)*	*Mean oblique error (D)*	*Distortion (%)*	
1.00	3.69	16.26	2.26	20.05	
0.70	1.03	13.89	−0.11	13.45	Minimum curvature error
0.50	−0.27	12.65	−1.35	9.91	Minimum oblique astigmatism
0.00	−2.50	10.31	−3.70	3.05	
−0.30	−3.39	9.26	−4.75	−0.13	Minimum distortion
−0.40	−3.36	8.95	−5.05	−1.07	

Using these expressions, ray tracing programs can be written to derive the oblique astigmatism and curvature error. For steeply curved surfaces, a small change in p has a significant effect upon the optical performance of a lens. Thus Table 7.5 illustrates the optical effects of changing the front surface of a +14.00 DS lens from spherical to various aspherical forms, while the rear surface remains spherical and of constant power.

It will be apparent that all three major aberrations cannot be reduced to zero at the same time. Astigmatism reaches a minimum with a p_1 of 0.5, curvature error or mean oblique error (MOE) is at a minimum with a p_1 of 0.7, and distortion is minimized with a p_1 of −0.3. Using two aspheric surfaces would not improve matters (Katz, 1982). So which design would be chosen in this case? Up until the 1970s the traditional design approach had been to minimize curvature error or oblique astigmatism, the design being little different at this power. However, lenses such as the Welsh Four Drop showed that flatter lenses with effectively lower values of p_1 giving low amounts of astigmatism could be very acceptable. Although the lens in Table 7.5 with −0.3 p_1 has appreciable oblique astigmatism and curvature error at 35° off axis, it also has low distortion. In addition, what is not apparent from the table is that the lens will be much better in appearance than the others as the front surface is flatter. The field of view will also be wider as a result of the lower prismatic effect at the edge of the lens. The fact that the visual acuity is worse at the edge has not been found to be a disadvantage, as wearers learn to overcome this by turning their head so that the visual axis passes through the centre of the lens where there is good visual acuity.

Although the post-cataract lens market was the main area for the use of aspherical surface spectacle lenses up till the 1980s, this market has now reduced in the developed world as a result of the use of intra-ocular implants after surgery. However, aspherical surface lenses are now being used in low power lenses (up to ±6.00 D) in order to provide reasonable optics in lenses of shallow form. This concept was proposed by Jalie (1980) for both positive and negative lenses, although the greatest benefit is to be found in positive powers.

Classification of aspheric lenses for aphakia

Conic surface lenses

Conic surface lenses have a surface geometry that can be described by the equation:

$$x = \frac{\dfrac{y^2}{r_0}}{1 + \sqrt{1 - p\left(\dfrac{y^2}{r_0^{\,2}}\right)}} \qquad \textit{Equation 7.04}$$

These are typically used for aspheric lenticulars, where the effective optical aperture is normally 42 mm. Full aperture lenses have been available in the past, but with a very restricted uncut diameter.

Polynomial surface aspherics

Polynomial surface aspherics are a variation on conic surface lenses, developed in the 1960s when designers used more complex surface equations to attempt more control over the optical performance (see, for example Davis and Fernald, 1965). These can be considered as conic surfaces modified by further terms, for example:

$$x = \frac{\frac{y^2}{r_0}}{1 + \sqrt{1 - p\left(\frac{y^2}{r_0^2}\right)}} + Ay^4 + By^6 \quad \textit{Equation 7.07}$$

These lenses are optically indistinguishable from conic surface lenses in most cases.

'Zonal' aspherics

'Zonal' aspheric lenses are not really aspherics at all, but are blended intersecting spherical curves of greater radius of curvature as distance from the pole increases, which behave as a pseudo-aspheric surface. This type of lens was first developed by Welsh (1978) in the 'Four Drop' lens.

In theory the smoothest curve would be obtained by using intersecting offset curves (Figure 7.15); however, this would give rise to very large changes in tangential power at the intersection of the zones (Smith and Atchison, 1983). In practical lens forms the coaxial construction is used (Figure 7.16). Although the change in tangential power, and thus increased oblique astigmatism, at the edge of each zone is still clearly apparent with this design (Figure 7.17), this is not noticed by wearers of this type of lens.

One benefit of this zonal type of construction was that it enabled lenses to be produced that were flatter in appearance than conic full aperture lenses, while typically having an uncut diameter of 58–60 mm, compared with 54–56 mm for the conic lenses.

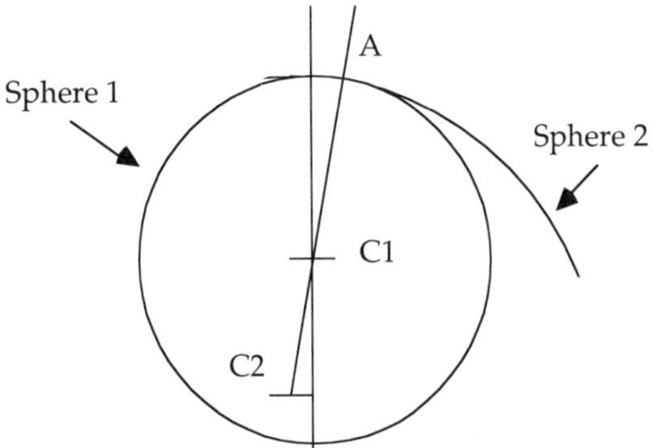

Figure 7.15. An offset zonal aspheric lens, showing the smooth curve that would be created by using curves with intersecting centres of curvature.

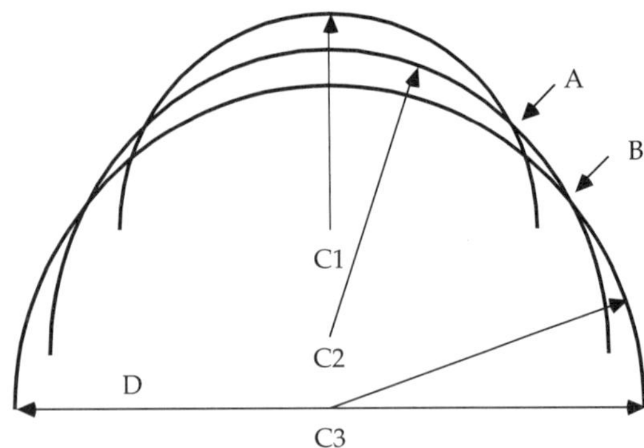

Figure 7.16. The coaxial construction commonly used in zonal aspheric lenses.

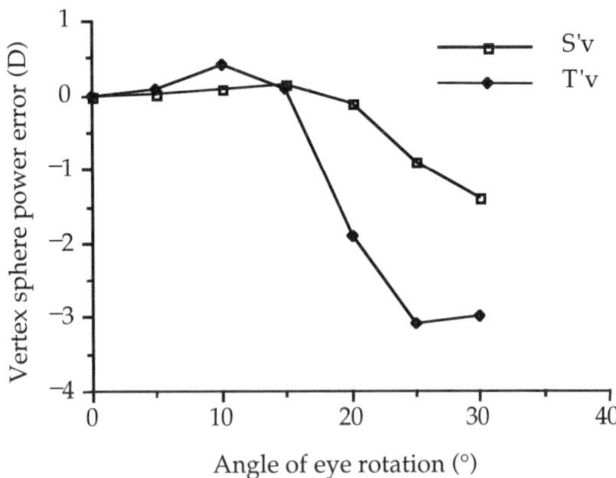

Figure 7.17. Sagittal and tangential powers of a coaxial zonal aspheric lens as the eye rotates away from the optical axis of the lens. Note that oblique astigmatism (the difference between the tangential and sagittal powers) increases markedly at the edge of the intersecting zones: at 15° of eye rotation, the eye would be looking through point A of the lens in Figure 7.16.

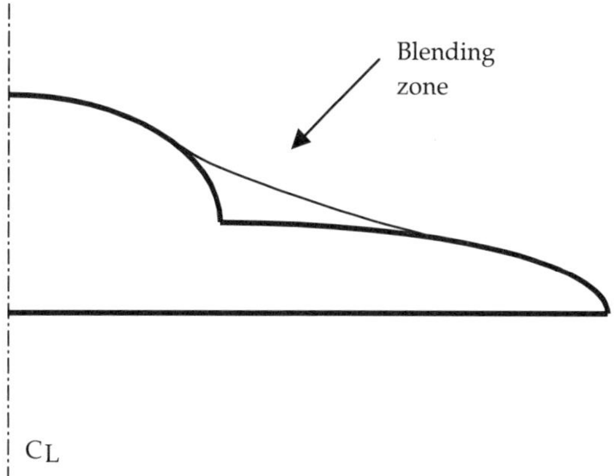

Figure 7.18. A blended lenticular lens. The lens consists of a central portion with the required vertex power and spherical curvature, and a low powered or plano carrier portion. The two portions of the lens are blended together to give a gradual change in curvature between the two sections.

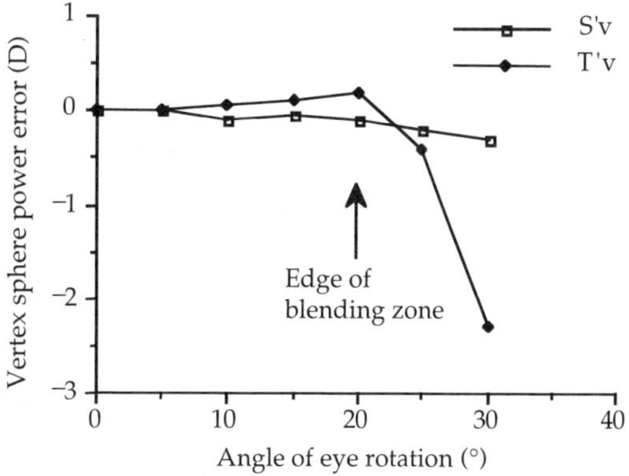

Figure 7.19. Sagittal and tangential powers of a blended lenticular lens as the eye rotates away from the optical axis of the lens. Note that oblique astigmatism (the difference between the tangential and sagittal powers) increases markedly at the edge of the central portion of the lens as the eye enters the blending area.

Blended lenticulars

Blended lenticular lenses grew out of the requirement for ever-increasing diameters for high positive power lenses, but without the cosmetic disadvantage of the lenticular construction (Figure 7.18). These lenses made uncut diameters of 66–67 mm available, but with the disadvantage of poor acuity in the blending area, where the curve is ground for purely cosmetic reasons to blend together the central powered portion and the unpowered carrier lens. Lenses of this type are sometimes described by polynomials of the form:

$$x = \frac{\frac{y^2}{r_0}}{1 + \sqrt{1 - p\left(\frac{y^2}{r_0^{\,2}}\right)}} + Ay^4 + By^6 + Cy^8 + Dy^{10} \qquad \text{Equation 7.08}$$

Such lenses are designed to give good visual acuity for eye rotations up to 25° off axis (Figure 7.19).

Aspheric lenses for high myopia

Tscherning's ellipse (Figure 7.11) shows us that lenses free from oblique astigmatism can be manufactured with spherical surfaces up to approximately –22.00 D, and up to even higher powers in high refractive index materials. Thus the vast majority of negative prescriptions can be made in an adequate form to give reasonable optics without the necessity of using aspherical surface lenses. The problem with high minus powers of large edge thickness still remains, so that a few designs have appeared for high myopia in aspherical form. Bettiol *et al.* (1980) patented a lens where the front surface was concave on axis, but convex in the periphery (Figure 7.20). Other designs have concentrated on a blended lenticular-type construction. Such designs can use a smaller effective aperture compared with equivalent plus power lenses as the peripheral prismatic effect gives an enhanced field of view (Figure 7.20).

Low power aspheric lenses

The patent of Jalie (1980) demonstrated how very shallow form meniscus lenses in low (up to ±6.00 D) plus and minus powers could be given acceptable off-axis optical performance if one surface was made aspherical. Jalie suggested that the front surface of plus lenses and the rear surface of negative lenses should be in aspherical form, the other surface being made spherical or toroidal depending on the prescription. The first lenses utilizing this concept were made in 1.6 refractive index glass, and were available in both positive and

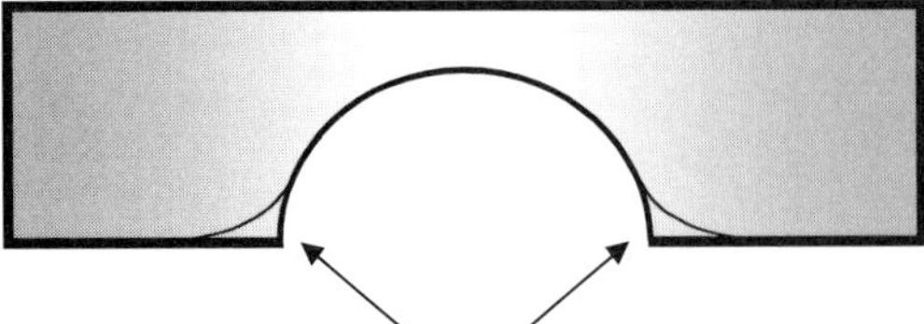

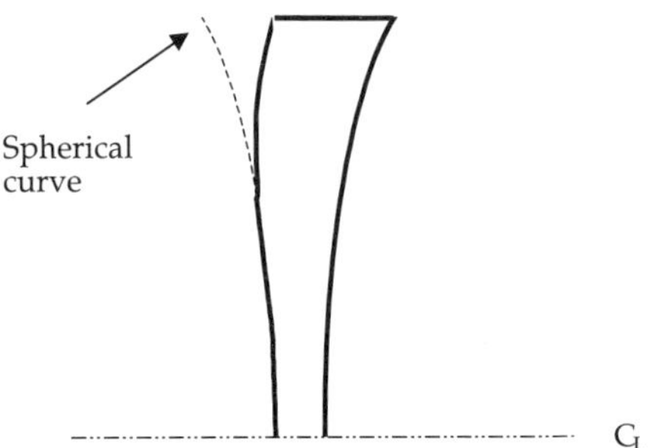

Figure 7.20. Examples of lens designs for high myopia. The upper portion of the figure shows a negative blended lenticular lens. The lower portion of the figure shows a lens with an aspheric front surface curvature. Both lenses are designed to minimize the edge thickness of the highly negative lens.

negative powers. However unlike Jalie's patent, the front surface of the minus lens was made aspheric. This was presumably because the ophthalmic industry is mostly only equipped for the manufacture of concave toroidal surfaces.

Although aspherical minus lenses have the benefit of a small reduction in edge thickness compared with their spherical equivalent, the biggest benefits are undoubtedly in plus power lenses where a substantial improvement in appearance can be achieved because of the flatter front surface in aspherical form. Thus the majority of lenses currently used in aspherical low powers are positive.

It must be emphasized that the aspherical surface is used primarily to improve appearance and reduce weight, and does not give improved optics over what is possible with the optimum spherical meniscus form. In Table 7.6, lens forms are given for both +3.00 DS and –3.00 DS lenses with spherical and aspherical front surfaces, the rear surface being spherical in all cases. Note that the first of the two spherical forms ($p_1 = 1$) in each case give lenses with minimal curvature or mean oblique error (MOE), while the second gives a form with minimal oblique astigmatism (AST). The third form in each case is a much flatter form meniscus, but still with a spherical front surface, while the fourth lens is a front surface hyperboloid aspheric. The distortion in percentage (DIST) is not, however, improved by using an aspherical surface in these examples. The minus form aspheric lens requires a very high value of p_1 because the front surface is a very shallow curve.

Examples of the off-axis power errors of two commercially produced aspheric lenses are shown in Figures 7.21 and 7.22, these being +6.00 DS and –6.00 DS BVP respectively. These lenses, as with many others of this type, are made in higher refractive index materials to further improve the cosmetic advantage. It should be emphasized that there are other constructions beside conic

Table 7.6 Spherical and aspheric lens forms for +3.00 DS and –3.00 DS lenses. Calculations based on an eye rotation of 30°, centre of rotation distance of 27 mm, and a lens material of 1.6 refractive index

Lens power	*p1*	*p2*	*F2*	*t (mm)*	*MOE (D)*	*AST (D)*	*DIST (%)*
+3.00	1	1	–5.00	3.0	+0.01	+0.19	+3.47
+3.00	1	1	–7.00	3.0	–0.13	+0.04	+3.02
+3.00	1	1	–1.00	3.0	+0.47	+0.70	+4.66
+3.00	–10	1	–1.00	3.0	–0.08	+0.08	+3.58
–3.00	1	1	–7.00	1.5	–0.06	–0.21	–3.37
–3.00	1	1	–10.00	1.5	+0.12	–0.01	–2.56
–3.00	1	1	–4.00	1.5	–0.38	–0.56	–4.47
–3.00	350	1	–4.00	1.5	+0.05	–0.02	–3.82

p_1, front surface asphericity; p_2, rear surface asphericity; F_2, rear surface power; t, centre thickness; MOE, mean oblique error; AST, oblique astigmatism; DIST, distortion.

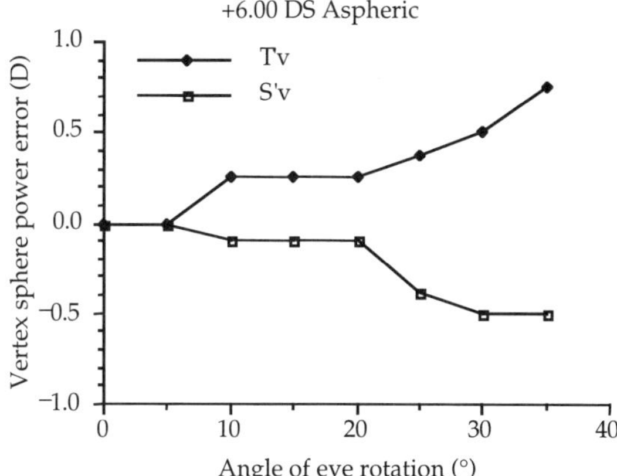

Figure 7.21. Sagittal and tangential powers of a low powered aspheric lens (+6.00 D) as the eye rotates away from the optical axis of the lens. Note that oblique astigmatism (the difference between the tangential and sagittal powers) increases away from the centre of the lens.

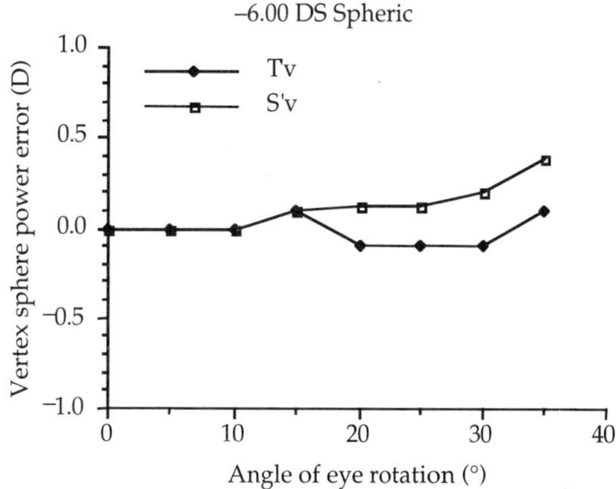

Figure 7.22. Sagittal and tangential powers of a low powered aspheric lens (−6.00 D) as the eye rotates away from the optical axis of the lens. Note that oblique astigmatism (the difference between the tangential and sagittal powers) increases away from the centre of the lens, but is not nearly as great as for the low powered positive lens.

surface aspherics. A form of blended lens with a peripheral flange of lower power is available for correction of hypermetropia. This lens is thinner and lighter than full aperture aspherics, but with the penalty of a slightly reduced optical aperture.

Aspheric toroidal surfaces

The majority of aspheric spectacle lenses are aspheric on only one surface – conventionally the front. The rear surface is then made spherical or toroidal, depending on the final prescription. This construction will only give good off-axis optical results if the lens is spherical or of low astigmatic power. If there is a large cylinder and hence a major difference in powers between the principal meridians, then the optics can only be optimized for one principal power. This is accepted for manufacturing convenience, as many aspheric front surface lenses are distributed in semi-finished form to optical laboratories who can only produce spherical or toroidal second surfaces.

To illustrate this problem, consider the lens shown in Figure 7.23. A +6.00 D lens has an aspheric front surface ($p_1 = -1$) and a shallow spherical rear surface ($p_2 = 1$). The sagittal (S′) and tangential (T′) values for a centre of rotation distance of 27 mm are plotted against angle of eye rotation. This shows that for distance vision the lens is commendably free from oblique astigmatism, this being only +0.10 D at 35° angle of eye rotation. As we would expect, the mean power does fall off as the eye rotates, so that instead of being +6.00 D at 35° the average of the sagittal and tangential powers is about +5.60 D.

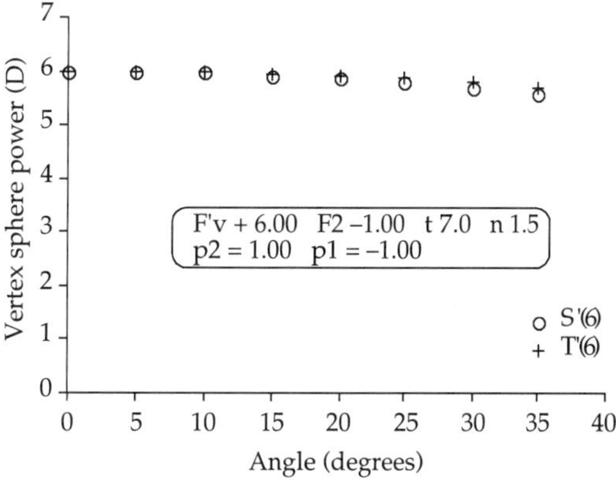

Figure 7.23. Sagittal and tangential powers of a low powered aspheric lens as the eye rotates away from the optical axis of the lens. The back vertex power of the lens is +6.00 DS and the lens is made with a spherical rear surface (*F*2 −1.00 DS; *p*2 = 1) and an aspheric front surface (*p*1 = −1). The lens is 7 mm thick and is made of material with a refractive index of 1.5.

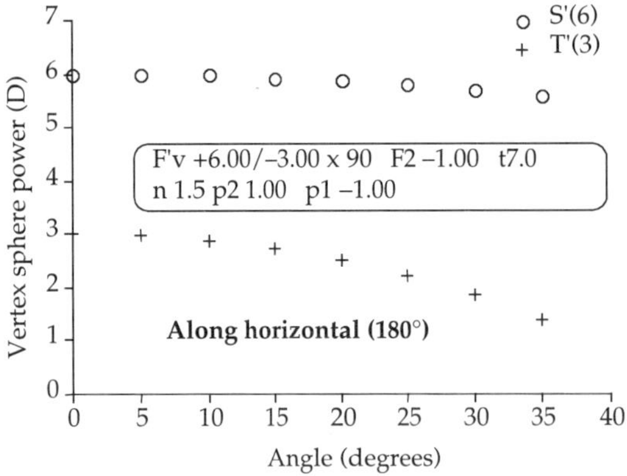

Figure 7.24. Sagittal and tangential powers for the same lens parameters as in Figure 7.23, except that the back vertex power of the lens is now +6.00 DS/−3.00 DC × 90. When considering angular rotation of the eye along the horizontal meridian, oblique astigmatism increases away from the vertex of the lens.

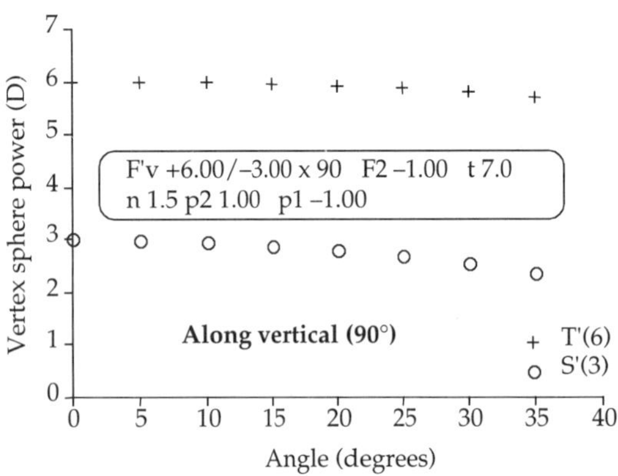

Figure 7.25. Sagittal and tangential powers for the same lens parameters as in Figure 7.24, angular rotation of the eye is considered along the vertical meridian. The oblique astigmatism is much less than in the horizontal meridian.

If we use the same aspheric front surface and centre thickness and now manufacture a lens with the final prescription of +6.00/−3.00 × 90, then the situation is very different, as illustrated in Figures 7.24 and 7.25. First consider the situation when the eye moves along the horizontal (180°). Here the tangential power is due to the +3.00 D meridian, and the sagittal power is due to the +6.00 D. At 35° the meridian power difference should be 3.00 D, the cylinder power, but it is actually 4.21 D. However, when looking vertically along the cylinder axis (90°) the situation is better, since the tangential power is due to the +6.00 D meridian and the sagittal to the +3.00 D meridian. In this case the oblique astigmatism is 3.32 D – only a 0.32 D error in cylinder power.

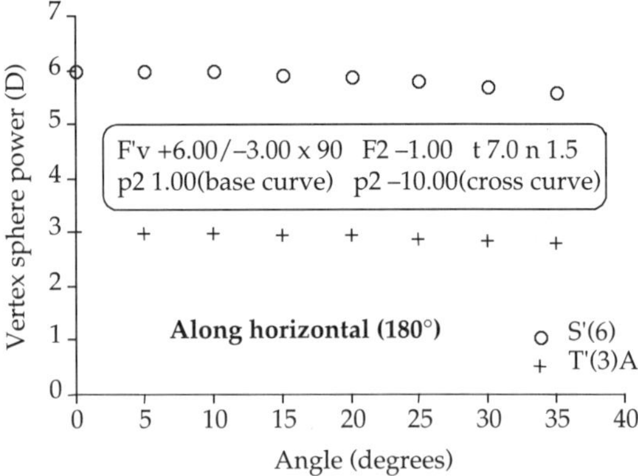

Figure 7.26. Sagittal and tangential powers for the same lens parameters as in Figure 7.24, except that the toric rear surface is also made in aspheric form. This has the effect of reducing oblique astigmatism in the horizontal meridian.

Thus the cylinder power will vary considerably depending on the direction, as well as angle, of gaze. A solution to this problem is to make the cross curve on the toric surface of aspheric form – sometimes known as an 'atoroidal' surface. It is also possible to make both curves of the toroidal surface aspheric if required. Figure 7.26 shows the effect of making the cross curve aspheric on the rear of cur theoretical sample lens. The toroidal surface is now spherical on the base curve ($p_2 = 1.00$), but hyperboloidal in form along the cross curve. At 35° off axis, the cylinder power is now 2.82 D rather than the required 3.00 D, but is much more acceptable at only a −0.18 D error.

In summary, aspheric lenses that are used for astigmatic prescriptions can benefit from using an aspheric toroidal surface when the prescription cylinder reaches high values.

Choosing and fitting aspheric lenses

Choosing

Lenses over +7.00 DS BVP can be made with better optical performance by using an aspheric form rather than spherical. Which of the lenses to choose in this group will depend on the priorities of the wearer:

Priority	*Lens of choice*
Thinnest	1.8 index glass aspheric
Thinnest and lightest	Aspheric CR39 lenticular
Largest uncut diameter	Blended lenticular
Widest field of good acuity	CR39 full aperture conic
Widest visual field	Zonal aspheric

Note that for all lenses, use of a high refractive index material with low constringence will tend to reduce the off-axis visual acuity as compared to materials having a high *V* value in the range 50–60, such as CR39 or crown glass.

In the high minus power range, the only advantage of the blended lenticular construction is cosmetic, as the optical performance in the blending area is poor. This type of lens does enable large aperture spectacle frames to be glazed with high prescriptions.

In the case of low power aspherics, there is a wide choice of materials, diameters and optical performance. It is difficult to predict which type of lens would be the best for any particular purpose.

Fitting

Aspheric lenses should be fitted more accurately than spherical designs, particularly in high power versions. Aspheric lenses only give a good optical performance when accurately centred. For general purpose prescriptions it is advisable to give some pantoscopic tilt to the frame and drop the optical centres, since the vision will be clearest when the line of sight is normal to the rear surface. Normal wearers will spend more of their time looking down rather than upwards. A rule of thumb is to drop the optical centres 2 mm for every 5° of pantoscopic tilt. Pantoscopic tilt is defined as 'the angle between the optical axis of a lens and the visual axis of the eye in the primary position, usually taken to be the horizontal' (BS3521, Part 1, 1991), and is shown in Figure 7.27.

It is a good idea to fit any lens over ±5.00 D to monocular centres rather than to a binocular measurement of interpupillary distance. Prism must *never* be induced by decentration of an aspheric lens, only by working on the rear surface. Before ordering aspherics it is worth checking carefully whether or not prism can be obtained in a required design.

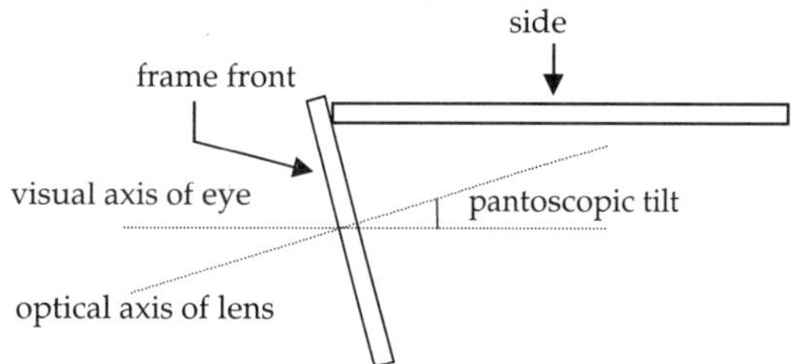

Figure 7.27. Pantoscopic tilt of spectacle front.

Low power aspherics for hypermetropes typically have much shallower rear surfaces than conventional curved form spherical designs, and these can cause annoying reflections to be apparent to the wearer. Therefore it is a good idea to add antireflection coating to these lenses (Chapter 10).

Checking aspheric lenses

Except in the case of uncut blended lenticulars, it can be very difficult to decide on casual inspection whether a lens is aspheric or not. Even if you are in possession of specialized equipment for tracing the surface or measuring the off-axis aberrations, the manufacturers only occasionally publish the design of their lenses, so it is difficult to determine whether the correct design has been supplied. A number of manufacturers are putting trademarks on the front surface of their lenses in the form of fine engravings.

The most straightforward qualitative test to detect whether or not a lens is aspheric is to use a lens measure in a sagittal section across the front surface (Figure 7.28). Spherical or toroidal surfaces will give a constant reading, whereas aspherical surfaces will vary in power.

Lenticular lenses

A lenticular lens is one in which the aperture containing the prescribed power is smaller than the frame aperture in which it is glazed. They are used for high power positive or negative presciptions where a full aperture

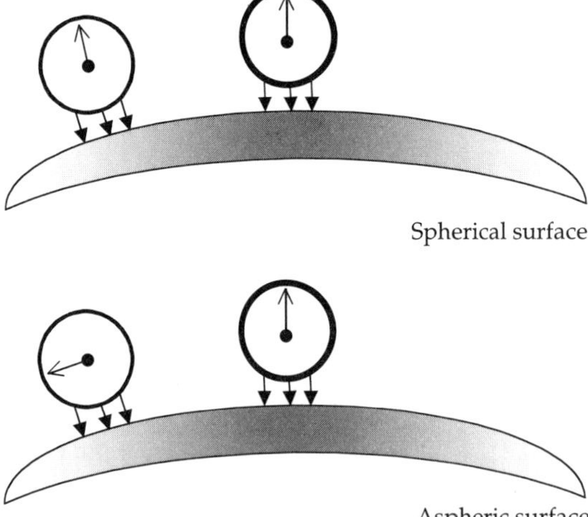

Figure 7.28. Identification of aspheric lens surfaces using a lens measure. The spherical surface has a constant radius of curvature across its surface, and hence will give a constant power reading in dioptres. The aspheric surface flattens towards the periphery, and will thus give a decreased power reading away from the vertex of the lens.

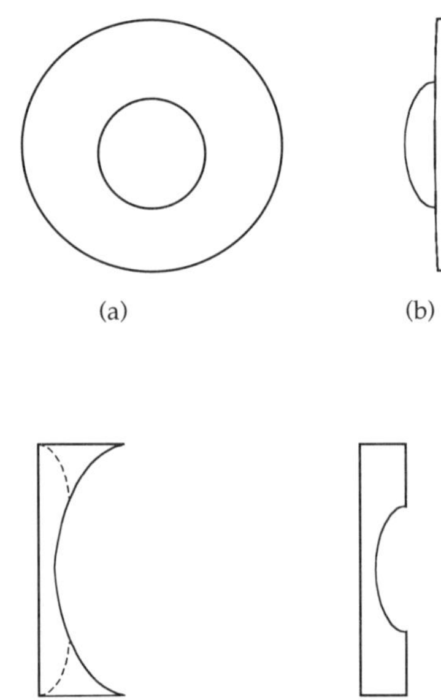

Figure 7.29. (a) Plan view of round aperture lenticular. (b) Cross-section cement positive power lenticular. (c) Flattened lenticular. Edge thickness reduced (to dotted line) by applying convex rear curve. (d) Plano margin lenticular.

lens would be too thick or heavy. Originally lenticulars were made in cemented form, where the prescription aperture was cemented to a carrier lens; however, the development of lenticular manufacturing technology closely followed that of bifocals (Chapter 8), so that solid and fused glass versions became available. Currently the majority of mass-produced products are moulded in plastics material.

Positive power lenticulars

The majority are now manufactured in solid form with a circular aperture in plastics material. The front surface of the aperture is commonly aspheric, and has a typical diameter of 40–42 mm. Spherical surface lenticulars commonly have an aperture diameter of 34 mm. Blended lenticulars are also available (see Figure 7.18) where a good cosmetic appearance is required with a large diameter.

Negative power lenticulars

There is a greater variety in design of negative lenticulars because some of these lenses can be manufactured on conventional lens prescription generators, unlike solid positive power lenticulars. The simplest design is the *flattened lenticular*, where a positive power is applied to the periphery of the rear surface in order to reduce the edge thickness. This process can be applied manually to give an aperture similar to the frame aperture (hand-flattened), or applied on a generator (machine-flattened), where a circular aperture is produced. Lenticulars are also produced for negative prescriptions by grinding a negative curve into a nominally plano lens (plano margin lenticular). As mentioned earlier, blended negative lenticulars are also manufactured (Figure 7.20).

Summary

In this chapter, the primary aberrations affecting image quality in spectacle lenses have been introduced. The significant aberrations affecting spectacle lens design are transverse chromatic aberration, oblique astigmatism, curvature and distortion. Different forms of lenses, such as best form lenses and aspheric lens designs, have been discussed in terms of their ability to reduce such aberrations.

Formulae

Formula	*Name*	*Equation number*
$\frac{n'}{s'} - \frac{n}{s} = \frac{n' \cos i' - n \cos i}{r}$	sagittal image position	7.01
$\frac{n' \cos^2 i'}{t'} - \frac{n \cos^2 i}{t} = \frac{n' \cos i' - n \cos i}{r}$	tangential image position	7.02
$y^2 = 2r_0x - px^2$	curve of conic section	7.03
$x = \frac{\frac{y^2}{r_0}}{1 + \sqrt{1 - p\left(\frac{y^2}{r_0^2}\right)}}$	conic section geometry	7.04
$r_s = [r_0^2 + (1 - p)y^2]^{1/2}$	sagittal radius of curvature	7.05
$r_t = \frac{r_s^3}{r_0^2}$	tangential radius of curvature	7.06
$x = \frac{\frac{y^2}{r_0}}{1 + \sqrt{1 - p\left(\frac{y^2}{r_0^2}\right)}} + Ay^4 + By^6$	polynomial surface geometry	7.07
$x = \frac{\frac{y^2}{r_0}}{1 + \sqrt{1 - p\left(\frac{y^2}{r_0^2}\right)}} + Ay^4 + By^6 + Cy^8 + Dy^{10}$	blended lenticular geometry	7.08

Exercises

Questions

1. A plano concave –10.00 DS back vertex power aspheric spectacle lens has a p_2 value of –0.5. If the refractive index of the material is 1.5, and centre thickness 1.0 mm, what is the lens diameter if the edge thickness is 6.0 mm?
2. A +6.00 D aspheric lens surface is made from material of refractive index of 1.8. If the p value is 0.3, what will be the sagittal and tangential surface powers at a point 25 mm from the axis of symmetry?
3. An aspheric +10.00 DS front vertex power lens has a plano rear surface. If the value of p_1 is zero, what will be the edge thickness for a diameter of 60 mm, if the centre thickness is 10.0 mm? ($n = 1.6$)

Answers

1. 45.3 mm
2. Sagittal power +5.93 D, tangential power +5.79 D
3. 2.5 mm

8

Bifocal and trifocal lenses

Bifocal lenses

The problem of presbyopia has exercised the minds of many spectacle lens designers throughout the ages. The ultimate goal has always been to give a spectacle wearer vision in presbyopia that compared with the state of affairs in pre-presbyopia. Full aperture near vision spectacles restricted the vision to near objects, and half spectacles were only suitable for those who were emmetropic in the distance.

The first recorded mention of bifocal spectacle lenses is a letter written by Benjamin Franklin in 1784 in which he describes a pair of spectacles incorporating such lenses. These were made by the relatively crude method of splitting a distance and a near lens, then mounting the top half of the distance and the bottom half of the near in the same frame (Figure 8.1). This approach is still in use for prescriptions that cannot be manufactured using mass-produced lenses, an example being where a large amount of prism is required at near but not at distance.

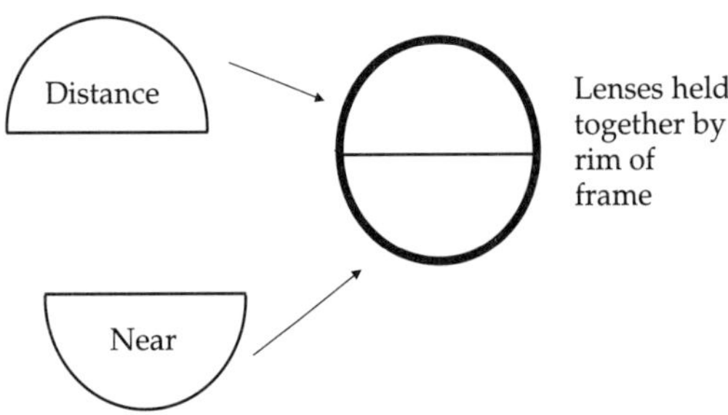

Figure 8.1. Schematic arrangement of a split bifocal, showing how the top half of a distance single vision lens and the bottom half of a near single vision lens are combined together.

Modern versions are improved cosmetically and mechanically by cementing the two lens halves together.

The split bifocal described by Franklin was not attractive, and was also expensive to manufacture. Another approach in the nineteenth century was to cement a small lens representing the near addition onto the distance prescription lens. Such lenses became known as cement bifocals, and again are still in use today (Figure 8.2). However, these lenses, although far better cosmetically than the split design, still suffered from the problem that segment could fall off due to poor cementing, and the segment was also prone to damage.

The obvious aim was to produce a one-piece lens that was good cosmetically, stable in construction, and yet economic for mass manufacture. Two such approaches were developed at the beginning of the twentieth

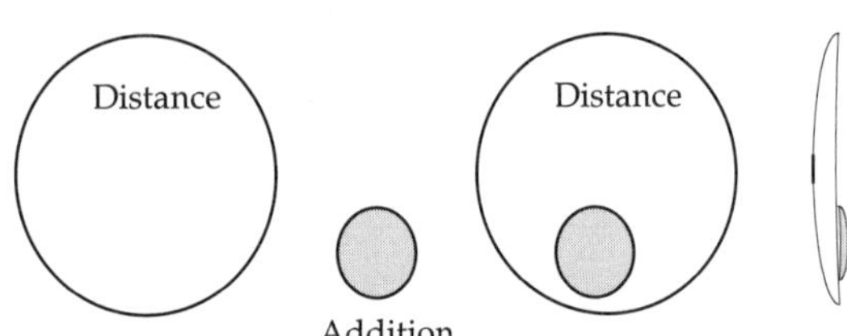

Figure 8.2. Cement bifocal with the segment cemented to the rear surface of a distance power lens.

century, fused and solid bifocals, and these still dominate the bifocal market.

Fused bifocals

Fused bifocals provide the extra positive power required at near in a presbyopic lens by incorporating a segment of high refractive index glass into the body of the distance lens (Figure 8.3). This was originally carried out by cementing the two components together, but subsequently it was discovered that the glass components could be permanently bonded by heat fusion.

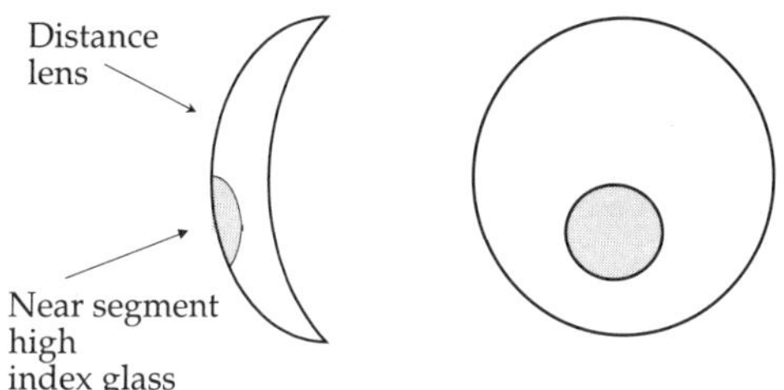

Figure 8.3. Cross-section and plan views of a circular segment fused bifocal.

The required addition depends on:

1. The refractive indices of the two glass materials
2. The contact radius between the components (the depression curve)
3. The curve worked on the segment side of the lens.

The two refractive indices are labelled n_c and n_f. The depression curve will have a radius of r_c, giving a power in air of F_c (Figure 8.4).

The front surface of the distance portion will have a surface power of F_1, and the front surface of the addition a surface power of F_3. The addition power is A. Thus:

$$A = F_3 - F_1 + F_{con}$$
$$= (n_f - n_c)/r_1 + (n_c - n_f)/r_c$$
$$= F_1(n_f - n_c)/(n_c - 1) - F_c(n_f - n_c)/(n_c - 1)$$
$$F_1 - F_c = A((n_c - 1)/(n_f - n_c))$$

Thus

$$F_c = F_1 - ((n_c - 1)/(n_f - n_c))A$$

As an example, consider a lens with F_1 of +6.00 D and refractive indices of 1.523 and 1.654 for n_c and n_f respectively. If an addition of +2.00 is required, then $F_c = 6 - (0.523/0.131)2 = -1.98$ D.

Fused bifocals have the distinction that they are the most 'invisible' of the types of bifocal mentioned so far when manufactured in the form described above with a circular segment.

At the present time the commonest type of fused bifocal is the shaped segment design, where a non-circular segment is used. Such lenses are manufactured by fusing a two-piece 'button' into the depression curve. One of the pieces of glass has the same refractive index as the major portion of the lens, and thus merges in the finished product, leaving a shaped segment (Figure 8.5). At one time many different shapes of fused segment were available, but currently these are limited to (Figure 8.6):

1. D segment
2. Semi-circular segment
3. B segment, sometimes known as a ribbon segment
4. Curved top D segment.

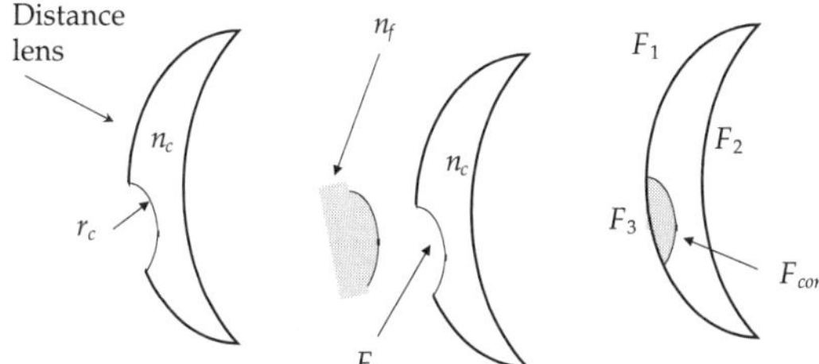

Figure 8.4. Stages in manufacture of a round segment fused bifocal.

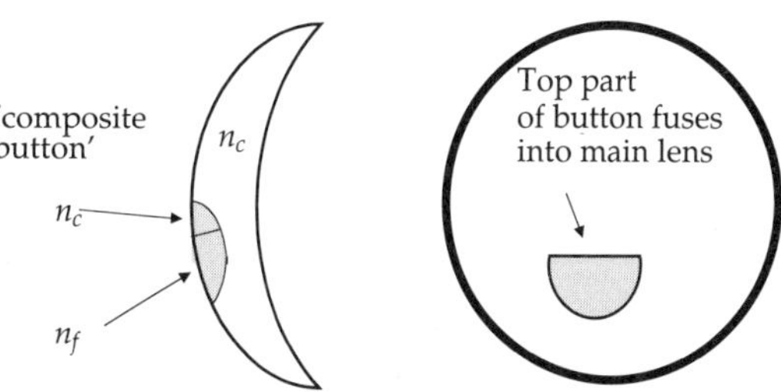

Figure 8.5. Straight top fused bifocal segment produced by using a composite button of two refractive indices.

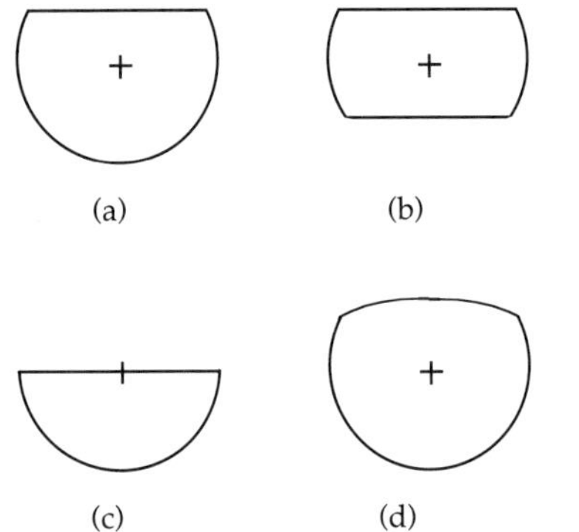

Figure 8.6. Fused bifocal shapes: (a) straight top (or D segment); (b) ribbon (or B segment); (c) semicircular segment; (d) curve top segment. Note that in each shape the cross indicates the geometric centre of the segment.

It is also possible to obtain similar shapes of segment in plastics materials, but in these cases the segment is produced as a solid bifocal rather than a fused.

Solid bifocals

The solid bifocal can be considered as a one-piece solid version of the cement bifocal. There are two basic types, *upcurve* and *downcurve*.

Upcurve bifocal

An upcurve bifocal is produced by grinding a negative power curve into a single vision lens, thus giving a negative addition (Figure 8.7). The segment contains the highest minus power, and is therefore the distance portion. This is the most straightforward type of lens to produce as a one-off item, but unfortunately it suffers from the fact that the near vision area is normally required to be smaller than the distance.

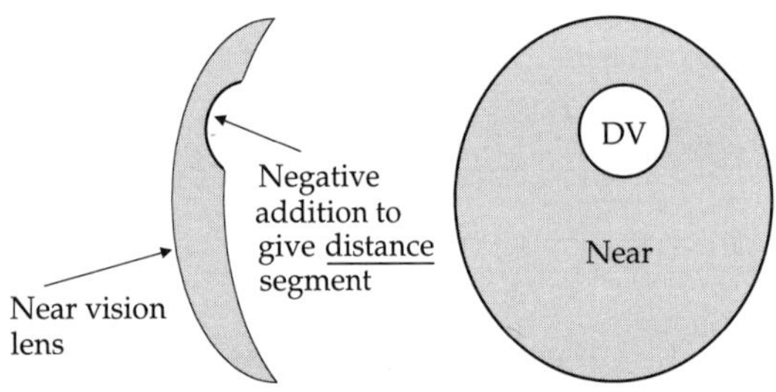

Figure 8.7. Cross-section and plan views of an upcurve solid bifocal.

Downcurve bifocal

The more popular downcurve bifocal is one where the segment stands proud of the main lens, and has a positive power addition in the segment. This is more complex to manufacture, as the lens is thicker in the near portion rather than the distance, and hence cannot be made from a single vision lens as with the upcurve (Figure 8.8).

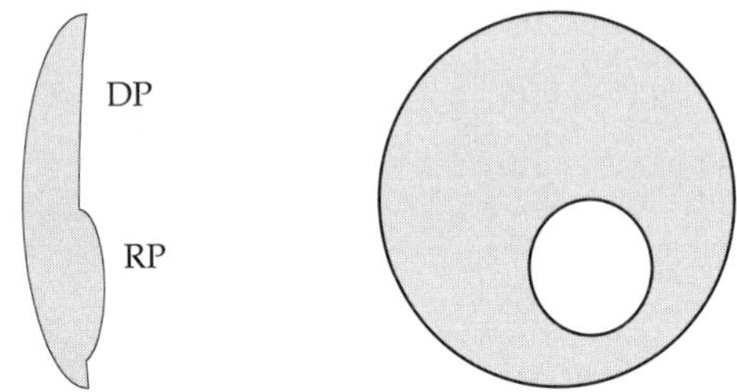

Figure 8.8. Cross-section and plan views of a downcurve solid bifocal.

Solid bifocals of this type are known as *downcurve* bifocals. In glass material the segment is positioned conventionally on the rear surface, but in plastics material it is generally incorporated into the front surface.

Solid bifocals with the appearance of one-piece Franklin split bifocals are also popular, these being called 'Executive' bifocals, a trademark of American Optical, or sometimes 'E style' (Figure 8.9). The advantage of this type of lens is the wide field of view at near, as well as improvement in optical quality.

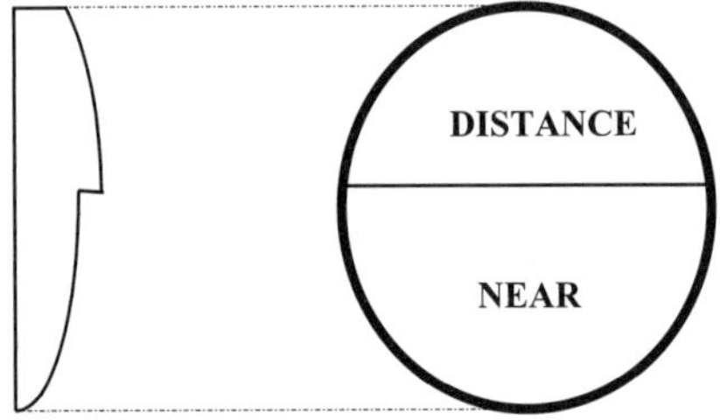

Figure 8.9. Cross-section and plan views of an E style bifocal. Note that distance portion has a finite thickness in order to give minimum thickness at near.

However, care must be exercised when using the E style as in hypermetropic prescriptions the lens can be excessively thick in the distance, particularly in high additions. This excessive thickness can be reduced to some extent by the careful use of *prism thinning* (see Chapter 9).

Solid-shaped segments are also manufactured in plastics material. The only problem with these designs is that there must be a ledge along any straight surfaces, which can accumulate dirt and is also prone to damage. At one time, round segment blended bifocals (generally known as *seamless* bifocals) were popular in the USA. These lenses have the least conspicuous segment of any bifocal, but are seriously compromised optically in the blending zone around the segment (Figure 8.10). They have been largely superseded by progressive addition lenses, which have a similar excellent cosmetic appearance but much improved optical quality.

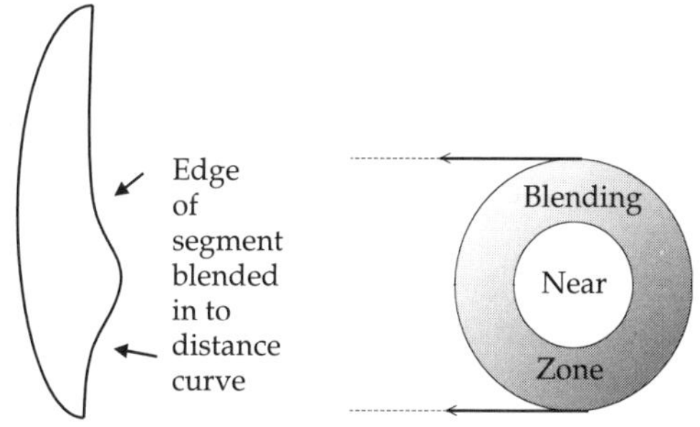

Figure 8.10. Cross-section through a seamless bifocal, with a schematic view of the segment, showing the annular blending zone.

Terminology

The description of bifocals is standardized in BS3521 (1991), Part 1. The more important terms are illustrated in Figure 8.11. Note that in a round segment the segment depth and segment diameter are the same, but that this is not the case in a shaped segment. Optical inset is rarely specified, as in most bifocals it cannot be independently controlled, being a function of the type of segment, geometric positioning, and the lens prescription.

In the case of large segment bifocals where the segment centre is not on the finished lens (Figure 8.12), geometric inset cannot be directly measured. However, the highest point of the segment will be directly over the geometric centre.

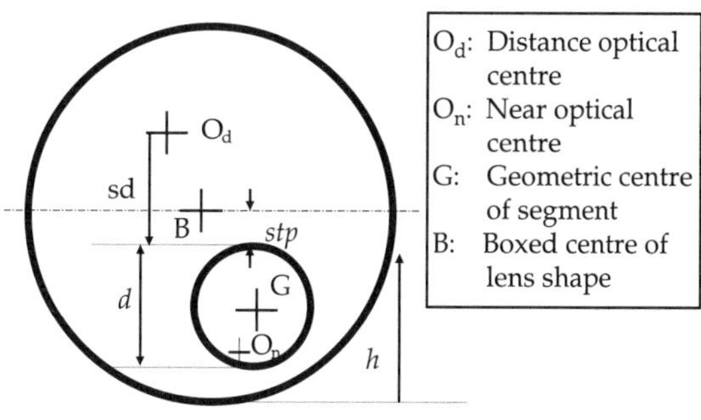

Figure 8.11. Bifocal terminology.

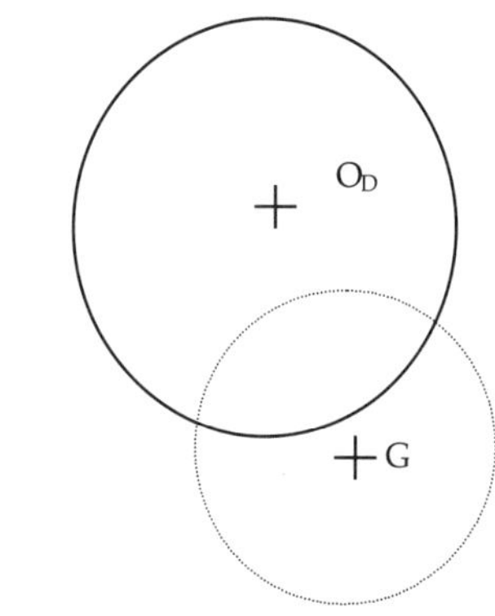

Figure 8.12. Large segment downcurve bifocal. Note that the geometric centre of the segment (G) is not on the lens.

Optical properties of bifocal lenses

Chromatic aberration

As a result of the fact that a bifocal segment is viewed through the edge of the distance lens, problems can arise due to transverse chromatic aberration arising from the distance vision prismatic effect. This is best illustrated by means of examples.

Consider a +5.00 DS distance lens, +3.00 addition, made with either a solid or fused segment, in crown glass ($n = 1.523$). The fused bifocal has a segment where $n = 1.654$. If we assume that the segments are both 22 mm in diameter, there is no geometric inset, and the segment top is 4 mm below the distance optical centre, then at the segment geometric centre the prismatic effect will be:

$P = cF$

$P = 1.5 \times +5.00$

$P = 7.5\Delta$ Base Up

This prism is due to the distance prescription only, as there will be no prismatic effect due to the segment. If the crown glass lens material has a constringence of 60, then the transverse chromatic aberration (TCA) at the segment centre is given by:

$\text{TCA} = (\text{F}/V).y$

$\text{TCA} = (5/60)1.5\Delta$

$\text{TCA} = 0.125\Delta$

This value will be the same for both the fused and solid bifocal.

However, if we consider another point 6 mm below the segment top (10 mm below the distance optical centre), then we have to consider the chromatic aberration induced by the segment as well. In order to make the calculations easier, Jalie showed that the fused bifocal can be split into three segments (Figure 8.13).

With very little error the above refractive indices give us a blank ratio of 4.00, thus the depression curve for a plano surface is:

$F_c = F_1 - 4.A$

$F_c = 0 - 4 \times 3$

$F_c = -12.00$ D

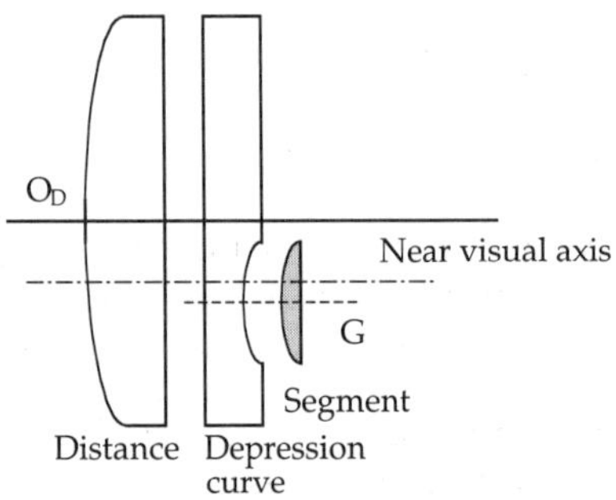

Figure 8.13. Schematic fused bifocal broken down into three components for the calculation of transverse chromatic aberration.

In order to give a +3.00 D addition, the high index glass segment must have a power of +15.00 D. We can now calculate the chromatic aberration along the near visual axis, lenses assumed to be thin.

At the point 10 mm below the distance optical centre, TCA due to:

1. Distance:
   $\text{TCA} = (F/V)y = (5/60) \times 1 = 0.083\Delta$ (Base Up)
2. Depression curve:
   $\text{TCA} = (F/V)y = (-12/60) \times 0.5 = 0.100\Delta$ (Base Up)
3. Segment:
   $\text{TCA} = (F/V)y = (15/30) \times 0.5 = 0.250\Delta$ (Base Down).

This gives a total TCA of 0.067Δ (Base Down).

In the case of the solid bifocal, this simply can be considered as a +5.00 D lens with a +3.00 segment on the rear, thus in this case the TCA would be calculated as:

1. Distance:
   $\text{TCA} = (F/V)y = (5/60) \times 1 = 0.083\Delta$ (Base Up)
2. Near:
   $\text{TCA} = (F/V)y = (3/60) \times 0.5 = 0.025\Delta$ (Base Down).

This gives a total TCA of 0.058Δ (Base Up).

There is very little difference here, but if the distance prescription were changed to –5.00 D then the base directions would be reversed for the distance component, giving totals of 0.233Δ for the fused and 0.108Δ for the solid.

Prismatic effects

As already discussed in relation to chromatic aberration, the optical properties of a bifocal suffer because the segment is positioned in the periphery of the main lens. This causes prismatic effects to be experienced by the wearer, which may cause problems in the cases of high prescriptions or anisometropia. Take as an example a –7.00 DS distance prescription, +3.00 D addition, 38 mm downcurve solid bifocal fitted with seg top 4 mm below the distance optical centre. If we assume that the wearer is looking through a point 6 mm below the segment top, what will be the prismatic effect?

Prism due to distance:

$P = cF = 1.0 \times -7.00 = 7.0\Delta$ Base Down

Prism due to addition:

$P = cF = 1.3 \times 3.00 = 3.9\Delta$ Base Down

Total: 10.9Δ Base Down.

This considerable prism would have some effect on visual acuity at near, particularly in low contrast conditions. To avoid such a situation, a smaller segment should be used. Note that large diameter downcurve segments always exert Base Down prism because the addition is positive, therefore are better used for hypermetropic prescriptions where the distance prescription will exert Base Up prism.

More serious problems occur in anisometropia, when a relative prismatic effect at near is induced. For example, if the above prescription is the right prescription of a pair of spectacles, and −2.00 DS is the distance prescription for the left eye, then the prismatic effects at near (N) will be as follows:

	R) −7.00 DS	*L) −2.00 DS*
Prism due to distance	7.0Δ BD	2.0Δ BD
Prism due to near	3.9Δ BD	3.9Δ BD
TOTAL	10.9Δ BD	5.9Δ BD
Relative prismatic effect	5.0Δ BD right	

This would certainly put the binocular system under stress, and steps must be taken to alleviate the prism, assuming that the patient is binocular to start with.

There are three basic choices to overcome this problem: unequal segment sizes, prism segment bifocals or bi-prism bifocals.

Unequal segment sizes

From Prentice's rule, the following expression can be deduced for round segment downcurve bifocals:

Difference in segment radii (in cm) × near addition = amount of relative vertical prism overcome

We have to assume one segment radius, as the expression only gives us the difference. The smallest segment is usually taken to be 22 mm (1.1 cm radius). Thus if we take the above example, with the unknown larger segment radius being x cm,

$(x - 1.1)3 = 5.0$

$3x - 3.3 = 5.0$

$3x = 8.3$

$x = 2.76$ cm

segment diameter = 55.2 mm

The larger segment would be placed in front of the more hypermetropic/least myopic eye, thus a combination of R) 22 L) 55 segments is required. This is not very good cosmetically, and is not a good solution in view of the better alternatives available.

Prism segment bifocals

These are downcurve solid bifocal lenses with the ability to incorporate prism into the segment, in 0.5Δ steps between 0.5Δ and 3.5Δ. The prism is produced by tilting the RP curve relative to the DP curve, which has the added effect of making the segment more visible. In general, Base Up prisms are better cosmetically, and should be used where possible. However, in this example since the amount of prism required is large (5Δ), the prism will have to be split between the two eyes, with 2.5Δ Base Up being placed in front of the right eye, and 2.5Δ Base Down being placed before the left.

Prism segments have been available in a number of different diameters at various times, but they are currently only available as 30 mm round, in glass.

Bi-prism bifocals

These lenses represent the best cosmetic solution to the problem of anisometropically induced prism. Also known as 'slab-off' bifocals, they can be produced from semi-finished lenses, or in plastic form some designs are moulded. One method of producing an E style lens from a standard semi-finished is shown schematically in Figure 8.14. Base Up prism is first worked across the whole of the rear surface. Next Base Down prism is worked on the distance curve of the front surface, on the top part of the lens only. This leaves a lens with zero prism at distance, and Base Up prism at near. The front surface

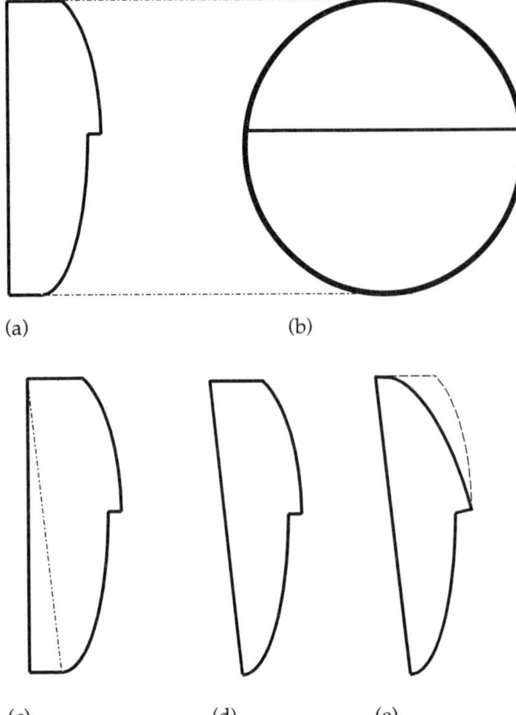

Figure 8.14. Stages in the production of an E style bi-prism bifocal from the semi-finished lens: (a) Semi-finished lens; (b) plan view; (c) base up prism applied across whole of rear surface; (d) lens with base up prism applied; (e) base down prism applied to front surface, distance only.

is worked on a 'D' segment so that the line between the two parts of the front surface coincides with the top of the segment. It is usually recommended that the minimum prism worked is 2Δ in order to obtain a clear dividing line between the two zones of the front surface.

Image jump

So far static prismatic effects have been described, but there can also be problems when the visual axis crosses the bifocal segment margin due to sudden change in prismatic effect. For example, in a conventional 22 mm solid or fused segment, the optical centre of the addition lens will be at the geometric centre of the segment. Thus as soon as the visual axis crosses the segment boundary there will be a sudden change of prism equivalent to the segment radius (cm) × addition. Thus a 38 mm segment with a +2.00 addition will give 3.8Δ at the segment edge, a 22 mm segment 2.2Δ, and so on. This prism is known as 'jump', as the effect on the wearer is for images to suddenly displace vertically at the segment boundary. The rule for downcurve segments is therefore that:

$$\text{jump (in } \Delta) = \text{the radius of the segment (cm)} \times \text{reading addition (D)}$$

For a shaped segment it is the distance from the top of the segment to the geometric centre, rather than the segment radius.

The effect of jump can be reduced to zero by placing the centre of curvature of the addition, the dividing line between the distance and near zones, and the centre of curvature of the distance curve, all in a straight line. The best known example of this is the 'Executive' lens, although semicircular segments are just as effective (Figure 8.15).

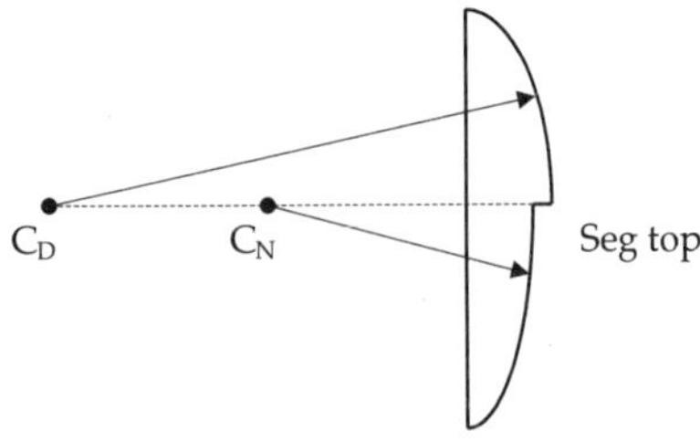

Figure 8.15. Condition for 'no jump' bifocal, showing that the centre of curvature for the distance curve (C_D), the centre of curvature if the near curve (C_N) and the segment top are all on a straight line.

Note that this will only eliminate vertical jump, horizontal jump still being present (Figure 8.16).

Field of view

The basic rule for field of view is that the larger the segment, the larger the field of view. However it is worth remembering that this field may be compromised by chromatic aberration at the periphery of the segment, and by aberrations, typically due to the major portion of the lens.

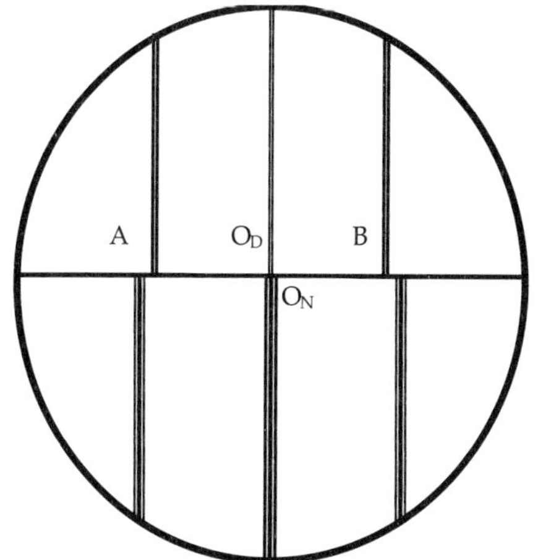

Figure 8.16. Lateral jump in an E style bifocal. Note that although a line through the optical centres of the lens will be undeviated, vertical lines at A and B show a lateral displacement at the segment top due to the unavoidable change in horizontal prism.

Verification of lens power in bifocal lenses

The distance portion of a bifocal lens is measured as if the lens were single vision by measurement at the centration point, which is usually the optical centre. The near addition must be verified by comparing the power through the segment *with a similar point in the distance part* (see Figure 8.17). The distance power at A must be subtracted from the near power at N to give the reading addition. Note that $A : O_D = O_D : N$.

It should be remembered that in bifocals the addition measured on the focimeter is really a *nominal* addition, as the measurement conditions do not simulate the lens in actual use. This is illustrated in Figure 8.18, which shows that the eye's visual axis passes obliquely through the lens for near vision, and that the effective vertex distance increases as the eye rotates downwards through an angle θ.

In BS 2738, Part 1 (1998) the conditions for determining the near addition power in front surface segment bifocals and varifocals are to take the difference in front vertex power measurements. How does this relate to the effective addition experienced by the wearer? For example, consider an Executive bifocal in CR39, with front surface powers of +8.00 D and +11.00 D. The finished lens has a centre thickness of 6.0 mm for distance, and 5.0 mm for near, and will have a near addition of +3.00 D by the BS method. If we further assume that the rear surface power is −2.00 D, this gives a BVP of +6.26 D for distance and +9.42 D for near. Hence if the addition is measured incorrectly by taking the difference in *back* vertex powers, then the measured addition will be +3.16 D. However, if we

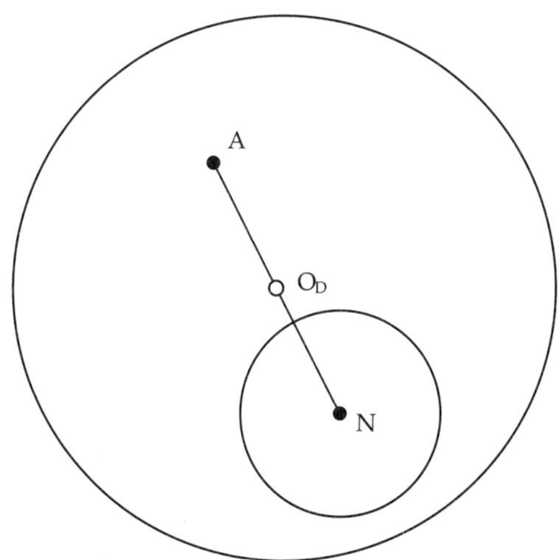

Figure 8.17. Theoretical verification points for a bifocal. Distance power should be verified at A and the near power at N. Note that position A may have been edged off a finished lens.

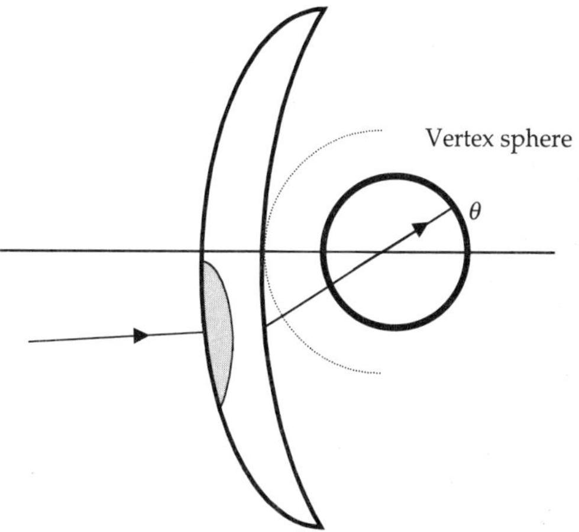

Figure 8.18. Effectivity of a segment in the 'as worn' position. Note that the eye is viewing obliquely through the segment, at an angle θ to the optical axis. As the eye looks further down, the vertex distance also increases.

carry out a ray-trace through the lens, for $\theta = 30°$, and a centre of rotation distance of 27 mm, then we find the following results:

Distance from optical centre (Front surface)	16.25 mm
Incident vergence	−3.00 D
Oblique astigmatism	+0.64 D
Mean oblique image vergence	+6.66 D
Thin lens image vergence = −3.00 + 9.42 =	+6.42 D
Thus overcorrection =	+0.24 D

Hence in this case the BVP measurement gives quite an accurate idea of the effective addition, but does not estimate the oblique astigmatism. It is difficult to give rule-of-thumb predictions of actual against measured (nominal) addition, but some lens manufacturers do publish this information for their own lenses. The best way therefore to measure the reading addition required for a bifocal is by over-refraction of an existing bifocal, but of course this procedure is not always possible.

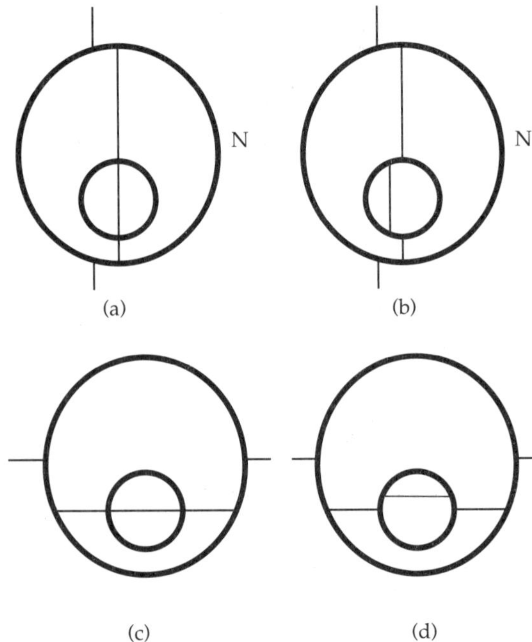

Figure 8.19. Effect of prism in downcurve solid bifocals. (a) No horizontal prism; (b) base in prism in segment; (c) no vertical prism; (d) base down prism in segment. In each case, the lens has been aligned so that the distance image is directed through the geometric centre of the segment.

Verification of prism in prism controlled bifocals

Prism segment bifocals

In these lenses, the prism incorporated must be compared with the prism induced by the distance prescription. The most practical way of measuring this is to neutralize any prismatic differences between the distance and near parts of the lens. In Figure 8.19, lens A shows a vertical line seen through the geometric centre of a 22 mm non-prism controlled segment, or alternatively a prism segment with no horizontal prism. Note that although there is displacement between the *object* line and the image vertical, indicating absolute prism, there is no deviation at the segment margin. In B a horizontal prism segment (Base In) is shown, giving a horizontal displacement in the segment of a line in the distance towards the segment centre. The segment centre is chosen as the reference point as this is the optical centre of the addition in a non-prism controlled lens. The task is to use trial case prism to neutralize the displacement in B so that the final view is as in A. A similar situation for vertical prism is shown in C and D, C being non-prism controlled, and D having Base Down prism in the segment. Note that this method only works if the lens is spherical, or the principal meridians are vertical and horizontal in an astigmatic lens. Where there is an oblique cylinder, a distorted image will be seen, and thus the cylinder must first be neutralized before the prism is assessed. It is not necessary to neutralize the spherical component.

Bi-prism bifocals

The prism can simply be assessed in a bi-prism shaped segment as shown in Figure 8.20, where the dividing line in the distance portion is placed mid-way across the focimeter aperture. This will give two vertically displaced focimeter images, the separation being the amount of prism worked on the segment, this being 3Δ in Figure 8.20.

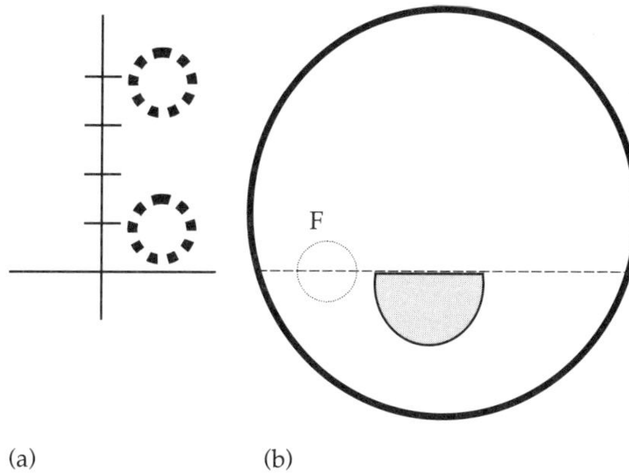

Figure 8.20. Verification of prism in a shaped segment, bi-prism bifocal. (a) An example where there are two focimeter images produced, corresponding to the distance power, vertically separated by the amount of prism incorporated, in this case 3Δ. (b) Right diagram shows the lens arranged so that the lens is placed so that the prism dividing line bisects the focimeter aperture (F).

Trifocal lenses

The first question to answer when considering trifocal lenses is why bother with them in the first place? This can best be illustrated by first considering an emmetrope with an amplitude of accommodation of 3.00 D. If we make a common assumption that two-thirds of this amplitude can be used for long periods of time, then the near addition required for near work at one-third of a metre is +1.00 D. Now if bifocals are used by this emmetrope, and ignoring any depth of field, then through the distance portion of the lens, if maximum accommodation is used, a range of clear vision from infinity to 0.33 m is possible. Using the near segment, the furthest point of distinct vision will be 1 metre and the nearest will be 0.25 m, again assuming that maximum accommodation is used. Note that the two ranges overlap.

However, if we now consider an emmetrope who has 0.75 D of accommodation, then by making the same assumptions as before, 0.50 D can be used for long periods, so that a +2.50 addition is (theoretically) required to see clearly at one-third of a metre. The clear ranges now become infinity to 1.33 m in distance, and from 0.40 m to 0.31 m at near. These ranges clearly do not overlap, so there is a zone between the distance and near where no clear vision is possible. The idea of a trifocal is partially or wholly to fill in this intermediate range with a reduced addition. Thus if a lens power for the intermediate of 50 per cent of near was chosen, which is a commonly used ratio, then the intermediate power would be +1.25 D, and the intermediate range of 0.80 m down to 0.50 m.

Thus trifocals are required by the older presbyopes who require higher additions. Construction of these lenses follows the same principles as bifocal lenses, so that they can be manufactured in split, cement, fused glass or solid forms (Figure 8.21). Note that fused glass designs require a segment with two refractive indices of glass in order to give the intermediate and near powers.

Although trifocal lenses have proved popular in the USA, they have largely been overtaken by the development of progressive addition lenses.

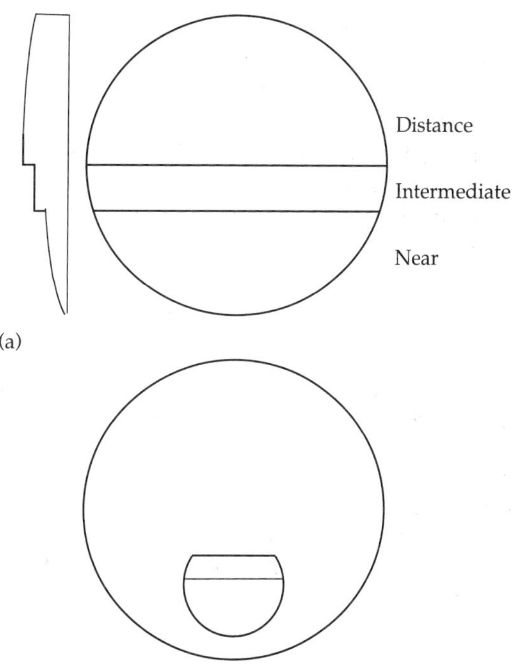

Figure 8.21. Two designs of trifocal lens: (a) E style trifocal; (b) D segment trifocal, manufactured in solid plastic or fused glass.

Guidelines for the fitting of bifocal and trifocal lenses

1. Distance prescription is centred as for a single vision distance lens.
2. The segments are inset so that the geometric centres of the segments coincide with the visual axes at near. Thus if the interpupillary distance (PD) is 64 mm and the separation of the visual axes in the spectacle plane while converged to the required fixation distance (near CD) is 60 mm, then each segment should have a geometric inset of 2 mm. Thus the distance optical centres will be 64 mm apart in the finished spectacles, and the geometric centres of the segments will be separated by 60 mm. Note that it is not possible to specify the position of the near optical centres in conventional fused or solid lenses.
3. The segment top of a bifocal should be positioned for an average fitting so that it is level with the lower limbus of the eye. This position may be higher if the wearer is only using the lenses for near work, or lower if the lenses are to be used predominantly for distance.
4. The top of the intermediate segment of a trifocal should be fitted level with the bottom of the pupil of the wearer. This position is quite critical. If the lens is positioned too high, it will interfere with distance vision. If too low, then there may be insufficient near segment in the frame to be useful.

Summary

In this chapter the major types of bifocal lens have been described, together with some of their advantages and disadvantages. The problems and compromises affecting all types of bifocal lens have been discussed, together with methods of overcoming some of the difficulties. A brief description is given of the rationale and use of trifocal lenses.

Exercises

Questions

1. A fused bifocal is required to have a +3.00 addition on a distance curve of +2.00 D. If the refractive indices are 1.600 and 1.700, calculate the power of the depression curve in air.
2. A fused bifocal with a front surface power of plano is manufactured with a +4.00 addition, and refractive indices of 1.523 and 1.654. If the segment diameter is 24 mm, what will be the centre thickness of the segment? (use approximate sag formula).
3. A bifocal with a distance prescription of –5.00/–2.00 × 90 has an addition of +2.00 D, with a 30 mm solid bifocal fitted so that the segment top is 5 mm below the distance optical centre. What will be the prismatic effect at the geometric centre of the segment?
4. If the distance prescription is R +1.00 DS L +2.00/+2.00 × 180, and the addition is +2.00 D, calculate the sizes of round segments required to eliminate relative vertical prism at a point 10 mm below the distance optical centres in each lens. Assume the smallest segment is 22 mm in diameter.
5. A prescription of R –10.00 DS L –10.00 DS, addition +2.00 D, also requires a prism of 2Δ Base in each eye for near only. If the geometric inset of each segment is 2 mm, calculate the amount of prism to be worked on to a prism segment bifocal to give this prescription.

Answers

1. –12.00 D
2. 2.2 mm
3. 10Δ Base Down
4. R 22 m L 52 mm
5. A prism segment is not required – conventional bifocals will give required prism.

9

Varifocal spectacle lenses

Introduction

Modern varifocal spectacle lenses have evolved over many years of development and can be considered as the ultimate progression from bifocals and trifocals. There are many ways in which a continuous power change can be given to a presbyope in order to aid near vision, these being divided into those devices that give a power change across the whole aperture of the lens, and those where the power change is limited to a small zone of the lens. So far all the commercially successful products have been in the latter group, the first group generally requiring some electrical, mechanical or hydraulic control system to vary the lens power. The history of variable power lens systems and progressive power lenses has been documented by Bennett (1970–1971) and Sullivan and Fowler (1988).

Lens systems

Deformable lenses

One of the simplest types of lens in concept, the central hollow cavity of a thin-walled lens is filled with fluid. When the fluid pressure is increased, the walls bulge outwards, giving an increase in positive power. The difficulties with this type of lens system include control of pressure, obtaining an even power change in two lenses, and leakage of the hydraulic fluid. Developments of this technique have used pressure on the rim of the lens to deform the surfaces, with the fluid being allowed to flow into the cavity from a reservoir.

Lens system with variable axial separation

Two lenses of equal and opposite power that neutralize one another when in contact will not do so if they are axially separated. This creates a positive power, which increases with lens separation (Figure 9.1). For example, a +10 D and –10 D pair of thin lenses will neutralize when in contact. However, if the lens separation is increased to 5.0 mm then the BVP of the combination will be +0.53 D, and if the separation is 10.0 mm the BVP will be +1.11 D. The major difficulty with this approach is in providing

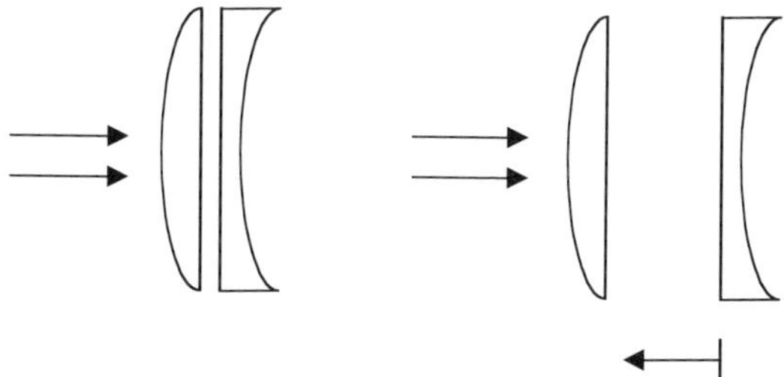

Figure 9.1. A lens system with variable axial separation. When in contact, the +10 D and –10 D lenses neutralize one another. When separated, the back vertex power of the combination becomes more positive.

a neat control system that is not unduly heavy or cosmetically disastrous.

Lens system with variable lateral separation

Unlike the system described above, where straightforward spherical lenses can be used, a lens system with variable lateral separation uses special elements (Figure 9.2) that neutralize one another when placed symmetrically (Figure 9.3), but provide variable power with lateral translation (Alvarez and Humphrey, 1970).

As before, these lenses suffer from the problem of mechanical control of the lenses, and the system has never been produced as a practical spectacle lens although it has been used in a refraction instrument – the Humphrey Vision Analyzer.

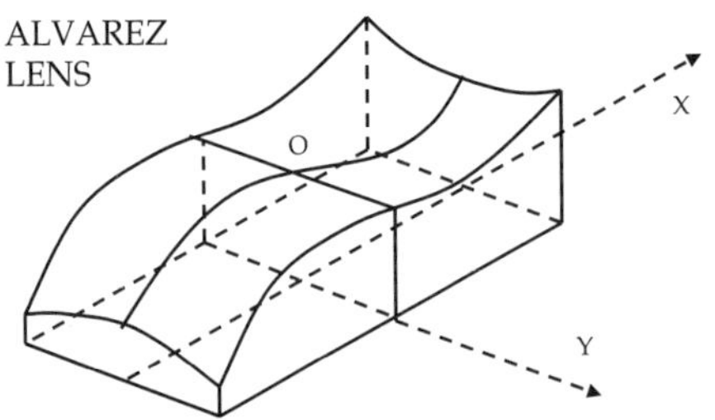

Figure 9.2. An Alvarez lens element. When two elements are combined and the lateral separation between them varied, the power of the lens is varied in a controlled manner.

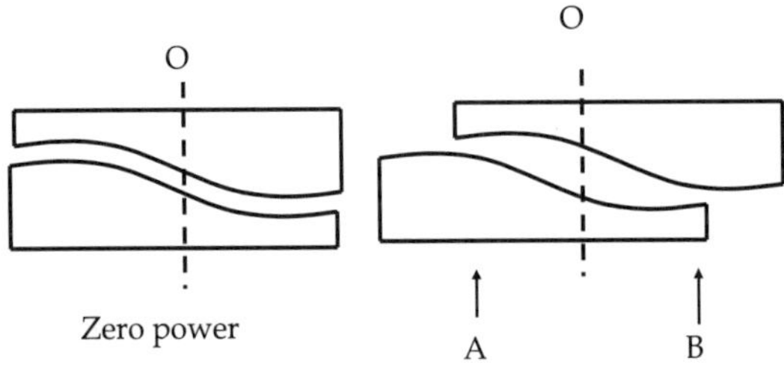

Figure 9.3. Alvarez lens elements used to produce a variable power spectacle lens by lateral separation. In (a) the lens elements are arranged symmetrically, providing a lens with zero power. In (b) the lens elements are offset. The lens thickness at A and B is greater than at O, and a negative lens has therefore been produced.

Lenses with variable refractive index

Liquid crystals have the property that their refractive index varies with applied voltage. This property has been suggested as a means for producing a variable power spectacle lens (Okada *et al.*, 1986), although no lens has been produced as yet. Unfortunately with liquid crystals the index also varies with the ambient temperature, and the lenses are affected by ultraviolet light.

Progressive addition lenses (PALs)

With progressive addition lenses the power varies across the aperture of the lens, the variation in power being fixed in a given design. This approach has produced all the commercially successful variable power lenses so far made, for two very good reasons. First, the lenses produced require no control mechanism to produce the power variation; secondly, the lenses appear very similar to single vision lenses, and hence are cosmetically very acceptable.

Progressive addition lenses – development

The first practical design for a progressive addition lens is generally accepted as that of Aves (1907). However, this lens used both front and rear aspheric cylindrical surfaces in order to provide a progressive power effect. The problem with this approach was that it would be very difficult to incorporate a cylindrical spectacle prescription. Thus the first commercially successful lens produced by the Société des Lunetiers in France in 1959 had a progressive surface on the front surface only, the rear surface being made spherical or toroidal depending on the requirements of the prescription.

Unlike the Aves lens, where the power varied continuously down the lens from top to bottom, the Varilux lens had two stable power zones, for distance and near vision, with a connecting variable power corridor down the centre of the lens. This central meridian is known as the umbilical meridian, and in order to give a spherical change in power the vertical and horizontal radii should match at any point down the umbilical meridian.

An idea of the mechanisms used and limitations imposed by the PAL concept can be gained by using the analysis of Volk and Weinberg (1962). Here a pair of aspheric cylinders is used, with axes mutually perpendicular in order to obtain a progressive power effect. Figure 9.4 shows the cross-section of a plane cylindrical element. The cylinder is a conic section, and note that the position of the centre of curvature (C) at any point will vary in the plane of the paper. If a section of this aspheric rod is taken and made into a plano-cylindrical lens, the radius of curvature decreases from top to bottom of the surface. Using the conic surface formulae from Chapter 7, the radius of curvature (r_s or r_t, for the sagittal and tangential radii of curvature respectively) can be calculated at any point which is a given distance (y) from the axis, using:

$$r_s = [r^2_0 + (1 - p)y^2]^{1/2} \qquad \textit{Equation 7.05}$$

$$r_t = \frac{r_s^3}{r_0^2} \qquad \textit{Equation 7.06}$$

The value of the paraxial radius of curvature is r_0, and the conic constant is p.

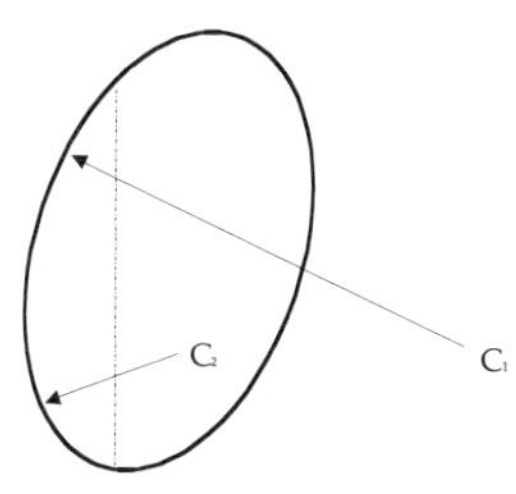

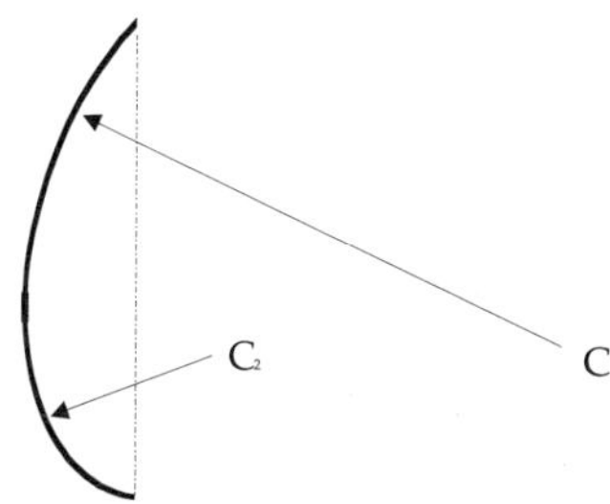

Figure 9.4. Aspheric cylindrical element. In (a) an elliptical cross section is shown. The radius of curvature decreases from top to bottom. In (b) a slice of the elliptical cylindrical rod is taken as a lens.

Figure 9.5a gives a schematic view of the power distribution in an aspheric plane cylinder, where the power variation is zero along the axis but varies from +1.00 D to +5.00 D perpendicular to the axis. If two such cylinders are combined with their axes mutually perpendicular, at 45° and 135° (Figure 9.5b), then the power distribution is as shown in Figure 9.5c. Note that this gives the power in cross-cylinder form, from which it is apparent that the power down the central portion of the lens is spherical but becomes increasingly astigmatic towards the periphery. Although this representation is schematic, it does indicate the problem of unwanted peripheral astigmatism inherent in the design of progressive addition lenses.

Many designs have appeared since the original Varilux was produced, improving the lenses by introducing the following features:

1. *Separate right and left lenses.* Original designs used a symmetrical construction that was swung nasally for convergence in each eye. The problem with this is that it increases the aberration level above the nasal horizontal line (Figure 9.6).
2. *Aspheric horizontal sections.* Original PAL designs used spherical sections, but these give a lens with very poor control of magnification and distortion, since as one looks down the lens, the power and also the magnification increase. Therefore, aspheric horizontal sections can be used, primarily to reduce distortion due to changes in peripheral power down the lens. Figure 9.7 shows a design concept where oblate ellipsoids are used in the distance zone, which increases the magnification towards the periphery of the lens. In the intermediate and near portions, progressively flatter prolate ellipsoid sections and hyperboloids are used in order to decrease the peripheral magnification resulting from the increase in power in the progression corridor.
3. *Different progression lengths.* Unwanted astigmatism in a progressive lens is dependent on the rate of change of power across the lens. By using a longer progression length the unwanted astigmatism is reduced, improving the visual acuity across the lens. Longer progression lengths

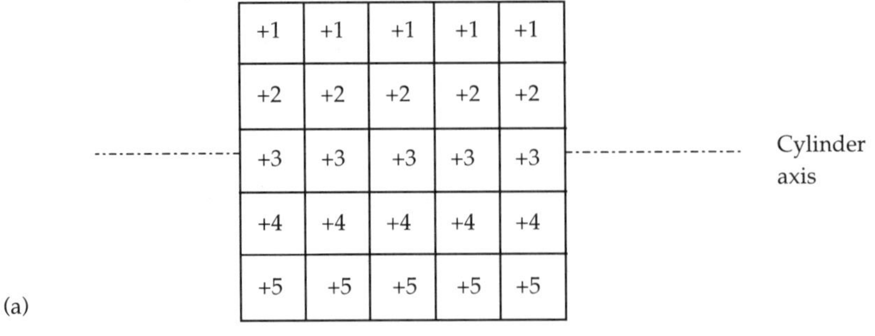

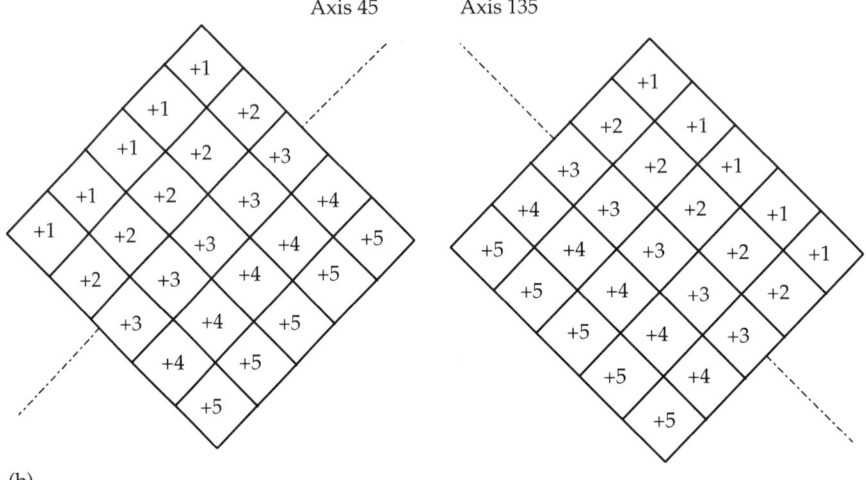

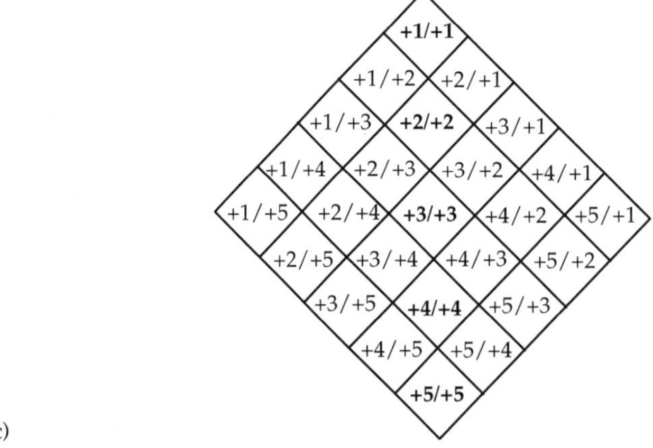

Figure 9.5. The use of two aspheric cylinders to create a progressive power effect. In (a) the individual aspheric plane cylinder is seen to have no power variation along its axis, being a constant +3 D. Perpendicular to the axis, the power varies between +1 and +5 D. In (b) two elements are shown, rotated to have axes at 45° and 135°, perpendicular to one another. The effect of combining these elements is seen in (c), where the power down the central umbilical meridian is spherical and increases progressively from +1 D at the top of the lens to +5 D at the bottom. Moving away from the umbilical meridian, the power of the lens is seen to become increasingly astigmatic towards the periphery. This is described as unwanted peripheral astigmatism, and compromises the quality of vision through the peripheral areas of the lens.

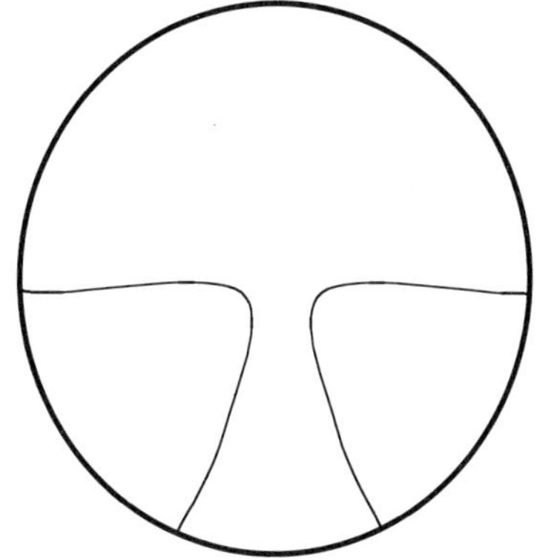

(a) Symmetrical progressive lens

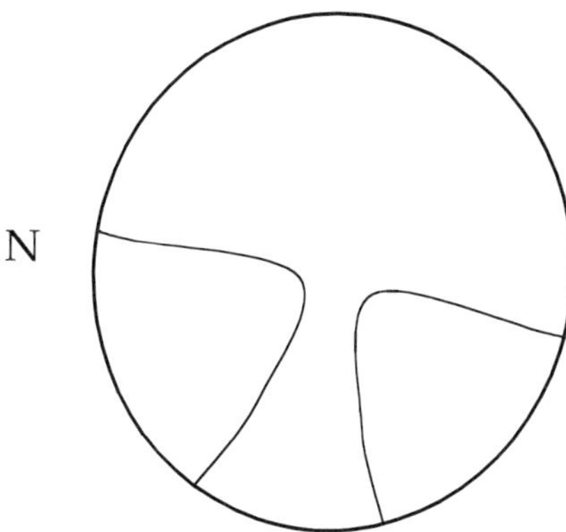

(b) Symmetrical lens rotated for convergence

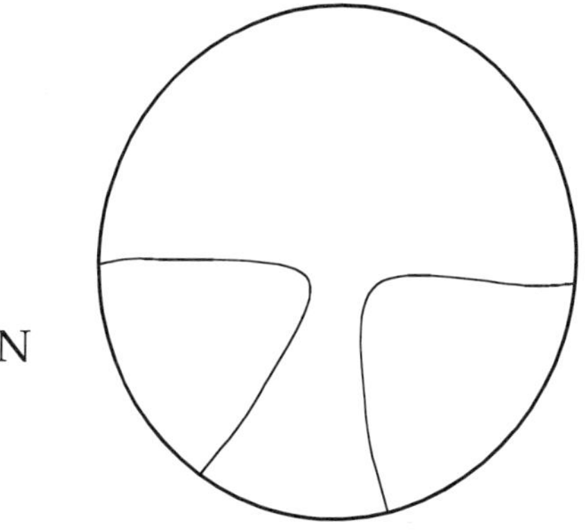

(c) Asymmetric design

Figure 9.6. (a) Schematic view of a symmetrical progressive lens design. The line indicates the limit of optimum visual acuity through the lens. Note the wide distance at the top of the lens, narrow intermediate in the middle, and wider near zone at the bottom. (b) The symmetrical lens rotated to allow for convergence at near, with compromised distance area. (c) Asymmetric design with no compromise at distance. N indicates the nasal side.

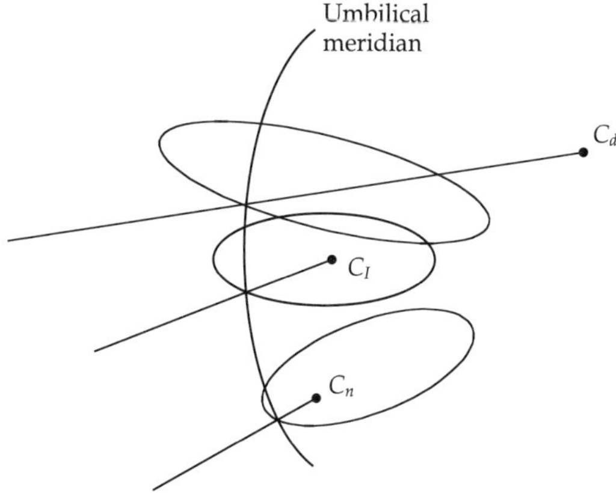

Figure 9.7. The use of aspheric sections in the construction of a progressive addition lens to control magnification and distortion. Moving down the lens there are two effects. First, the paraxial radius of curvature becomes shorter, giving increased power towards the bottom of the lens. Secondly, the asphericity of the surface changes, with the p value decreasing progressively down the lens. C_d, centre of curvature for distance; C_I, intermediate, C_n, near.

were only possible because of the fashion in many parts of the world for large aperture spectacle frames in the period 1970–1990. Thus in 1960 a large aperture spectacle frame would have had a 48 mm horizontal lens size, whereas when fashions changed values of 56–58 mm were not uncommon. In the late 1990s small aperture spectacle frames became fashionable again, which created a demand for lenses with shorter progression lengths.

4. *Development of non-standard lenses.* A number of designs have been produced over the years (with varying commercial success) that do not conform to the classical concept of progressive addition lens. Some examples of these include:
   a. Occupational progressive lenses – for example, a progressive lens with a 40 mm solid bifocal segment in the upper portion. This was originally designed for use by civil airline pilots, who at one time had to operate switches in the cockpit roof.
   b. Near vision lenses with enhanced depth of field – these are near vision lenses with a long progression extending upwards from the stable near portion, giving a small variation in power so that

the range of clear vision is extended compared with a single vision lens of the same power (Figure 9.8).

c. Bifocals with a variable power segment – these are bifocal lenses where the 'D'-shaped segment incorporates a progressive power change. The advantage of this construction is that, by removing the requirement for invisibility of the power change, the optics of the progressive zone can be improved.
d. Progressive power lenses for high plus prescriptions – these are blended aspheric lenticulars which incorporate a progressive power change. The progression is shorter than in conventional progressive lenses.
e. Progressive power lenses for viewing VDU displays – these are essentially progressive lenses with a long corridor, and small distance and near zones.

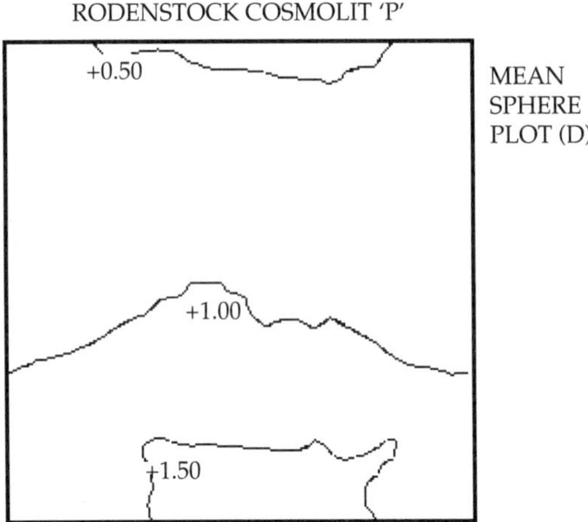

Figure 9.8. Mean power measurement of Rodenstock Cosmolit 'P' variable power near lens. (Values in dioptres, 40 × 40 mm plot, Fowler and Sullivan (1990) measurement method.)

Current lens design philosophies

The 'classic' progressive power lens can be summarized as having:

1. Stable (or nearly so) distance power in the top half of the lens
2. A stable reading area located in the bottom central area of the lens
3. A progressive power corridor joining zones 1) and 2)
4. Complete 'invisibility' of appearance, giving a single vision lens-type appearance.

This type of approach is popular because it overcomes two inherent disadvantages found in bifocals and trifocals: poor cosmetic appearance due to the segment, and lack of continuous power change between distance and near. Hence this type of lens has the widest appeal, as it can satisfy a number of requirements simultaneously. There are now many competing lens designs aimed at the 'general purpose' market. At one time it was common for manufacturers to have a specific design philosophy – for example, minimum surface astigmatism, or optimum visual acuity across the lens. In recent years, however, most lenses have become more of a compromise between the various concepts.

The terms 'hard' and 'soft' in relation to progressive lenses

The origin of the nomenclature 'hard' and 'soft' goes back to the early 1970s, when the first aspheric front surface lens (Varilux 2) was introduced. Among the features of this lens was the fact that the transition from distance power to the start of the progression was much smoother and less abrupt than in earlier lenses (Figure 9.9). One of the key benefits was that this made the lens less sensitive to small errors in vertical fitting position. This then gave rise to the term 'soft' to describe lenses with a gradual start to the progression, and 'hard' indicating the original type of progressive lens designs. The extreme of hard design is the bifocal, where the power changes from distance to near effectively instantaneously, and the ultimate 'soft' lens is one where the power changes across the whole aperture of the lens without any stable zones.

Over the years, the hard and soft descriptions have widened to describe lenses with certain groups of characteristics. For example, soft lenses will *tend* to have:

- Longer progression lengths
- Aspheric distance curves
- Small stable distance and near zones
- Low surface astigmatism.

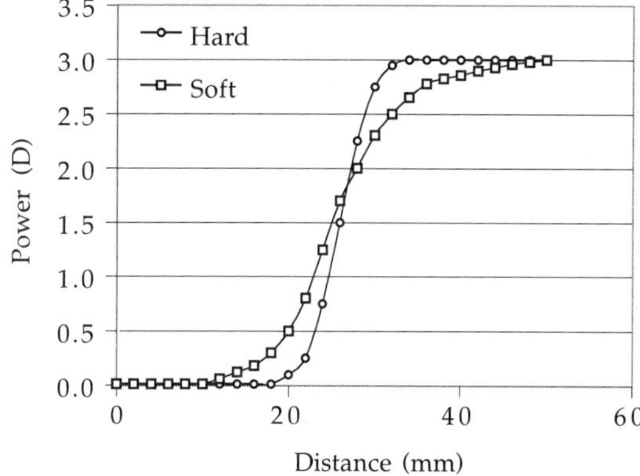

Figure 9.9. A comparison of the progression in 'hard' (circles) and 'soft' (squares) progressive lenses. The graph shows the power of the lens as a function of the distance below the distance fixation point. It can be seen that the progression in the 'hard' lens begins somewhat further down the lens than in the 'soft' lens, meaning that the 'hard' lens has a greater area of stable distance vision. The rate of change of power in the progression is much faster in the 'hard' lens than in the 'soft', and leads to a larger area of stable near vision in the 'hard' lens design.

By comparison, hard lenses will tend to have:

- Shorter progression lengths
- Spherical distance curves
- Large stable distance and near zones
- High surface astigmatism.

These features can be demonstrated in a number of ways. Figure 9.10 shows schematic astigmatism contour plots for two lenses, one hard and one soft. Note the lower level of surface astigmatism in the soft lens, and also that the top half of the hard lens is virtually free from surface astigmatism, indicating a larger area of stable distance power. The near area for the hard lens is also larger than that in the soft lens.

A further point to consider is the power of the addition. Because the distance from the stable distance zone to the stable near zone is virtually constant in most designs, the rate of change of power is going to be greater as the near addition power increases. Thus at low additions (for example +1.00 D), all designs will be quite soft.

It must be emphasized that labelling lenses as hard or soft is a relative description only. All general purpose lenses designed in the last 10 years can be considered soft compared to the original progressive designs. Thus making a list of current designs and designating some as hard and some as soft is meaningless, as there are no absolute standards of measurement. Manufacturers often now describe their varifocal designs as being 'add-based' or 'multi-designs'. An add-based varifocal design varies according to the power of the addition, whereas a multi-design varies according to the base curve of the lens, essentially meaning that the design varies according to the distance refractive error.

Comparison of progressive addition lenses

It is difficult to compare progressive addition lenses because of their complex aspheric

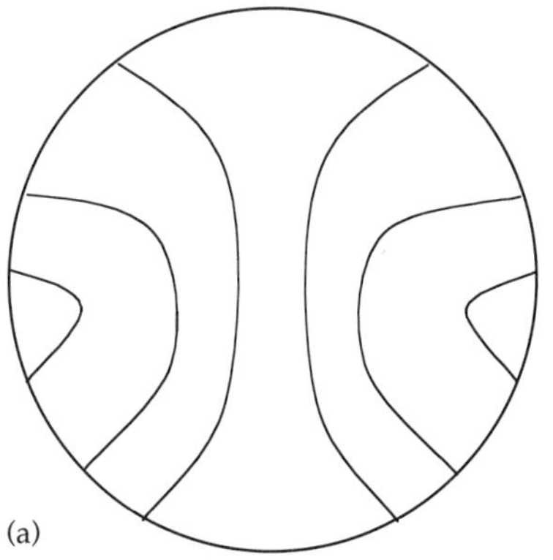

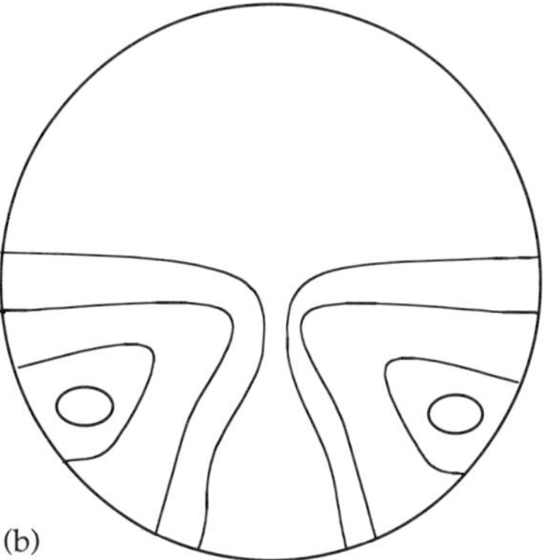

Figure 9.10. Schematic iso-cylinder plots for 'soft' progressive addition lens (a) and 'hard' (b). Note the spread of astigmatism into the distance of the 'soft' lens, and the increased astigmatism in the 'hard'.

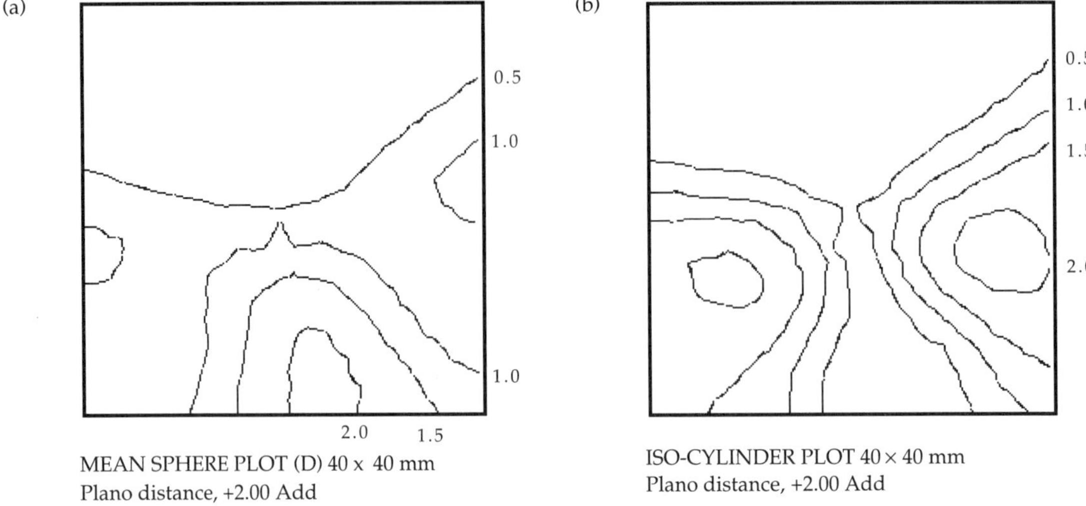

Figure 9.11. Contour plots of one design of modern progressive addition lens: (a) mean sphere; (b) iso-cylinder.

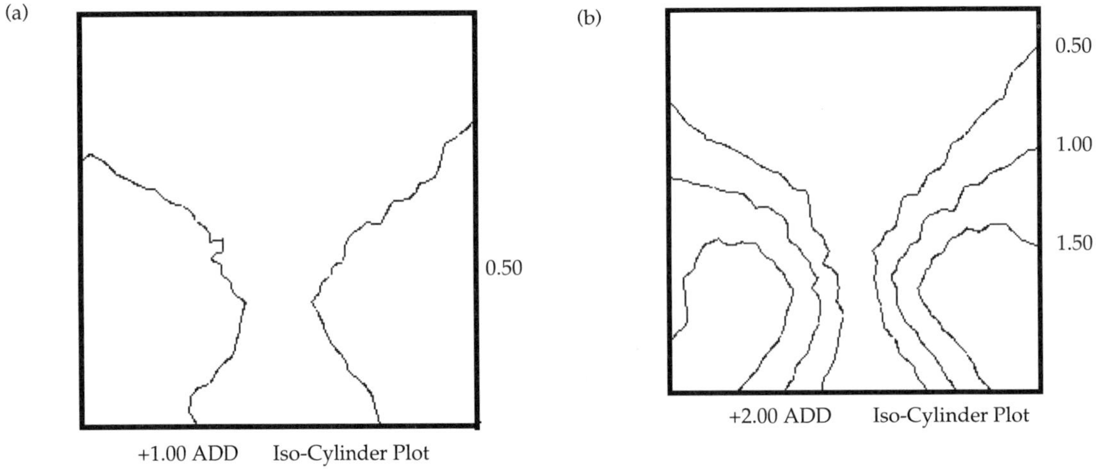

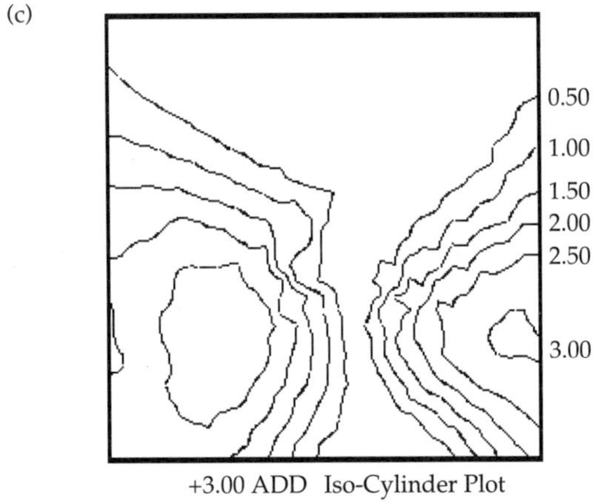

(a)

0.50

+1.00 ADD Iso-Cylinder Plot

(b)

0.50

1.00

1.50

+2.00 ADD Iso-Cylinder Plot

(c)

0.50

1.00

1.50

2.00

2.50

3.00

+3.00 ADD Iso-Cylinder Plot

Figure 9.12. Iso-cylinder plots for one design of progressive addition lens at three different additions: (a) +1.00; (b) +2.00; (c) +3.00.

surfaces. This is further compounded by the fact that it is difficult to predict the wearer response to the optical characteristics of a lens.

The commonest way of 'fingerprinting' a lens to give a broad idea of its characteristics is to produce contour plots. These are diagrams indicating areas of iso-cylinder or mean spherical power (Figure 9.11). For a realistic comparison, contour plots at additions across the design range must be viewed (Figure 9.12). Although these diagrams are useful for making basic classifications, they give no indication of the wearer acceptability of a given lens, for which clinical trials are essential.

Prism thinning

A feature of many progressive lens designs is the incorporation of vertical prism in order to reduce the thickness and weight of the lenses. Since the same amount of vertical prism is incorporated into both right and left lenses, there is no relative prismatic effect for the wearer. Figure 9.13 illustrates prism thinning in diagrammatic form. Note however that the universal incorporation of prism will not reduce the thickness in all prescriptions, as shown in Figure 9.14. In some instances, using prism will make the lens thicker.

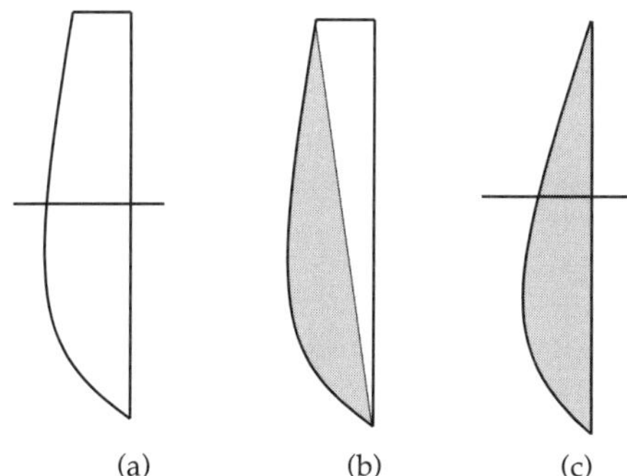

Figure 9.13. Prism thinning of a varifocal lens. (a) Side profile of a low-powered conventional progressive lens, with the distance portion essentially flat, and the radius of curvature shortening progressively in the lower part of the lens. (b) Base Down prism is applied to the lens in order to reduce the centre thickness, resulting in a lens as seen in (c). Since the same amount of Base Down prism is applied to both lenses, there is no relative prismatic effect.

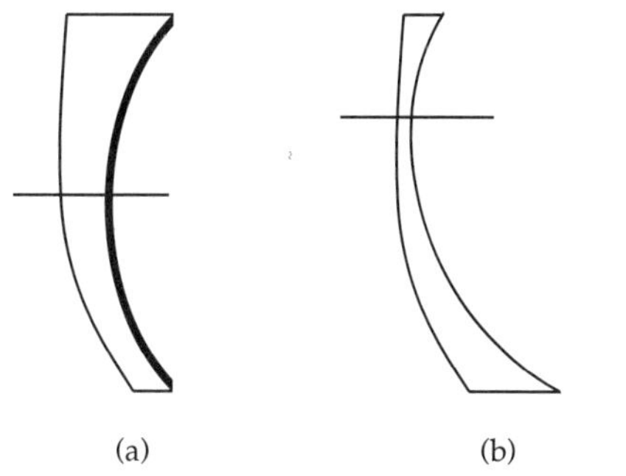

Figure 9.14. Cases where prism thinning of varifocals is not advisable. (a) Progressive lens with a negative prescription for distance and no prism thinning. The lens is fitted low, with the horizontal line indicating the prism reference point of the lens. The effect of adding a standard amount of prism thinning would be simply to move the thick edge from the top to the bottom of the lens. A small amount of prism thinning would be useful to equalize the edge thickness at the top and bottom of the lens. (b) Progressive lens with a negative distance prescription and no prism thinning, this time fitted high. The effect of adding Base Down prism in this instance would be to increase the thickness at the bottom edge of the lens. Base Up prism thinning would be of advantage here.

Identification and verification of progressive addition lenses

Although progressive addition lenses are now produced by many manufacturers, general purpose designs tend to use similar methods of identification. In Figure 9.15 a

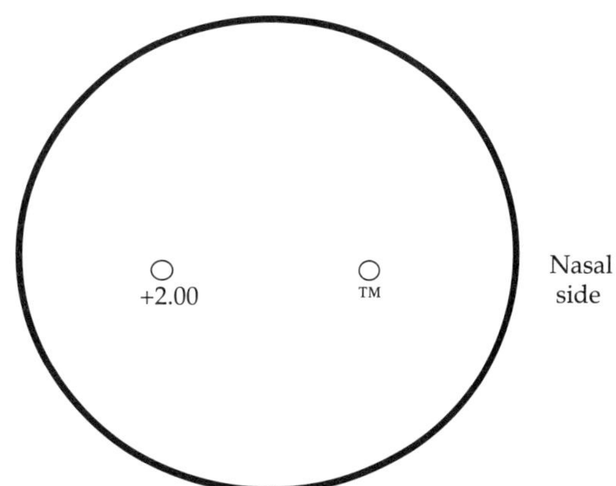

Figure 9.15. Permanent engravings on a progressive addition lens. The two engraved circles are placed 34 mm apart. On the temporal side the addition is engraved, and on the nasal side the manufacturer's marking is shown.

generic diagram of the faintly engraved identification marks found on the front of most lenses is shown. The two circles, 34 mm apart, indicate a horizontal axis through the geometric centre of the lens uncut. This axis will normally be placed parallel to the horizontal centre line of the frame. Note that other geometric shapes besides circles are also used. Beneath the nasal circle is a manufacturer's trade mark (TM), although this is not always present. Beneath the temporal circle is the reading addition in dioptres.

In order to indicate other landmarks on the lens, additional non-permanent markings are put on the front of the lens by the manufacturer (Figure 9.16). The distance vision power is checked at the 'horseshoe' marking (a), which is deliberately positioned well above the start of the progression. This is so that the power read will be stable and unaffected by the surface astigmatism due to the progression. In normal fitting, the cross (b) is placed in front of the pupil centre with the eye in the primary position. In the absence of any prism, the dot (c) indicates the optical centre of the lens. However, since most progressive lenses incorporate some prism thinning, the prismatic power read at this point will be the combination of the prism thinning plus any prescribed prism. Unless prism has been prescribed, the prismatic power at (c) should be the same in each lens, often about two-thirds of the addition in Base Down prism. The near vision power is checked at (d), within the stable near vision portion of the lens. As the progressive power surface is on the front surface of the lens, the addition should be measured as the difference between distance and near front vertex powers, as with front surface bifocals (Chapter 8).

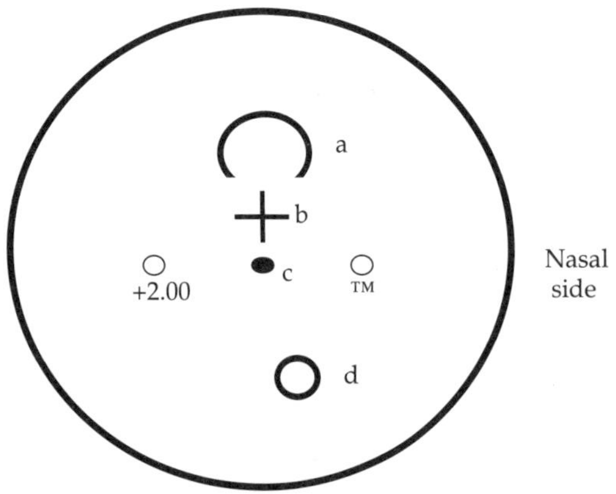

Figure 9.16. Additional temporary markings on a progressive addition lens. a, distance prescription checking point; b, fitting cross; c, prism reference point; d, near prescription checking point.

These temporary markings are purely for use in glazing and subsequent verification and are, of course, removed before the lenses are supplied to the patient. The markings can be easily removed with an appropriate solvent, but care should be taken because some lens and frame materials are damaged by acetone. Most manufacturers supply templates so that these verification positions can be subsequently re-marked, using the engraved circles as reference points. The engraved circles can be most easily found again by holding the lens front surface down against a dark background, with light directed onto the rear surface of the lens.

Fitting progressive lenses

Accurate positioning of progressive lenses is essential for their successful dispensing. Progressive lenses should also be fitted using the actual frame to be dispensed, adjusted to fit the patient, and with particular attention paid to the correct adjustment of the pantoscopic angle (Chapter 7). The centre of the patient's pupil should be marked when the person is fixating a distant object, and monocular PDs and vertical distances from the horizontal centre line recorded. The lenses must be fitted monocularly because of the narrow progression corridor.

In higher additions, the corridor is narrower than at low values (Figure 9.12). Many lenses have a fixed value for convergence at near, and if the patient does not converge by this value, then problems may arise at near vision due to non-optimum parts of the lens being used. Therefore for high additions (> +2.50) it may be necessary to fit to the near centration distance, and accept any induced prism caused by not having the lenses located normally for distance.

To fit the majority of progressive lenses, the patient's pupil centre should be at least 22 mm above the lower rim of the frame. This depth is required to ensure that the full progression length and sufficient stable reading area are present in the glazed lens. Some designs are available with slightly shorter progressions that require only 18 mm depth below the pupil, and these can be used in cases where the frame is too shallow for conventional progressive designs.

Summary

In this chapter, the design of lenses with variable power for dispensing to the presbyope has been discussed. Of those designs suggested, only the progressive addition lens has proved commercially viable. The design of these progressive addition (or varifocal) lenses has been discussed, as well as the differences between design philosophies in this type of lens, and, finally, identification, verification and fitting of varifocal lenses.

10

Tinted and treated lenses

Tinted lenses

Tinted spectacle lenses are used for a number of purposes. First, they are used to reduce glare across the visible spectrum, which requires a tint that absorbs radiation across the required range. Secondly, tints are used to protect against harmful radiation, which as far as general purpose spectacle lenses are concerned means the non-visible ultraviolet (UV) wavelengths. Thirdly, some wearers want a tint purely for the cosmetic appearance, with no particular concern regarding the transmission requirements. Manufacturers of tinted lenses, particularly those intended for protection against sun glare, often try to address all three requirements, so that a lens cuts down glare, gives good UV protection and also has a cosmetically pleasing colour.

The method of incorporation of a tint into a lens will depend on the lens material.

Glass lenses

Solid glass tints

Solid glass tints are produced by introducing tinting materials into the glass mixture at the time of manufacture. For example, oxides of iron and manganese give green and pink colours respectively. Only very small amounts are needed, and the mixture must be very carefully controlled in order to give consistent results. As the tinting material is distributed evenly throughout the lens material, this means that the tint density will depend on the lens thickness. In Figure 10.1, the transmission through a 3 mm sample lens is illustrated, where the material has a basic transmission of 80 per cent per mm. Ignoring reflections, 80 per cent is transmitted after 1 mm, 80 per cent of 80 per cent (or 64 per cent) is transmitted after 2 mm, and 80 per cent of 64 per cent (or 51.2 per cent) is transmitted after 3 mm. Such calculations are quite straightforward; however, in reality the situation is often more complex than in this simple example, and transmission is rather more difficult to calculate. It is therefore better to use optical density for the calculation of lens transmission, as densities can be

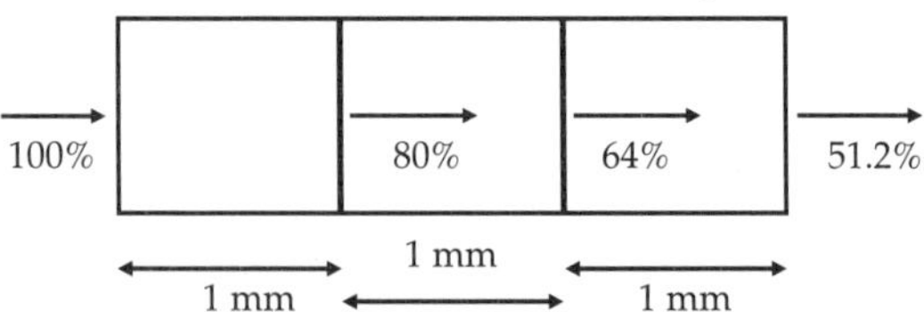

Figure 10.1. Transmission of light through a 3 mm lens with transmittance of 80% per mm; 100% of the light is incident on the front lens surface. After travelling 1 mm through the lens, 20% of the light has been absorbed and the remaining 80% is transmitted. After travelling a further 1 mm through the lens, 80% of the light available at the beginning of the lens section is transmitted, or $0.8 \times 0.8 = 64\%$ of the initial incident light. After a further 1 mm of travel through the lens, the proportion of light exiting the lens is $0.8 \times 0.64 = 51.2\%$ of the original incident light.

Table 10.1 Example calculations using optical density. In example A, a 2 mm thick lens with a tint of 25 per cent transmission is shown to have an optical density of 0.60. If the lens thickness increases to 3 mm, this lens will have a transmission of only 12.5 per cent. Examples B and C demonstrate further changes in transmission seen when reducing (example B) or increasing (example C) lens thickness

Solid tint transmission		*Example A*	*Example B*	*Example C*
Transmission (%)	TR	25.00	64.00	80.00
Transmission (max 1.0)	T = TR/100	0.25	0.64	0.80
Thickness (mm)	*d*	2.00	2.00	1.00
Density	D = log(1/T)	0.60	0.19	0.10
New thickness (mm)	*n*	3.00	1.00	3.00
New density	ND = D × *n*/*d*	0.90	0.10	0.29
New transmission (Max 1.0)	NT = 1/(10 ND)	0.1250	0.8000	0.5120
New transmission (%)	NTR = 100 × NT	12.50	80.00	51.20

arithmetically manipulated. For example, a lens 3 mm in thickness will have an optical density three times that of one 1 mm thick. The relationship of transmission to optical density is given by:

$$\text{Density} = 1/(\log T) \qquad \textit{Equation 10.01}$$

where T is the transmission and is given on a scale of zero to 1.0, where 1.0 is equivalent to 100 per cent. Examples of calculations using optical density are shown in Table 10.1. For simplicity, these calculations assume that there is no loss of transmitted light from reflection. Note from the table how a lens with the same optical density becomes less transmissive with increasing thickness (examples A and C). In practical terms, a solid tint will appear darker in thicker portions of the lens. For example, the edges of a highly negative lens, the centre of highly positive lens, or the higher powered lens of an anisometropic correction will appear more deeply tinted.

Glass photochromic tints

Glass photochromic tints are a special group of solid materials that change their tint density with the incident light, and also with temperature. Silver halide crystals doped with copper are mixed in with the glass at the time of manufacture, and in the borosilicate mixture used by Corning the photochromic process can be represented as:

$$Ag^{+} + Cu^{+} + UV \rightarrow Ag + Cu^{++}$$

The silver halide crystals are activated by UV radiation and blue light of the visible spectrum within the range 300–400 nm, with maximum activation caused by light of wavelength 355 nm. The influence of this radiation causes a colloid of metallic silver to appear. Once the UV light is removed the reaction reverses, promoted by heat. In practical terms, therefore, a photochromic lens darkens in sunlight and fades when not exposed to sunlight. A typical glass photochromic response curve is illustrated in Figure 10.2. Note that the fading (recovery) rate is much slower than the darkening. The fading and darkening of photochromic lenses are affected by heat – the lenses go darker in colder conditions, and are less effective in hot climates. The time course is also thickness-dependent, with thicker lenses taking longer to return to the faded state. Transmittance values should therefore be quoted for a specified temperature (preferably 25°C) and thickness (usually 2 mm) to allow comparison between materials.

Photochromic lenses can be classified according to their transmittance in the faded (maximum transmittance) and darkened (minimum transmittance) states (BS 7394, Part 2, 1994), as shown in Table 10.2. For

Table 10.2 Classification of photochromic lenses (BS 7394, Part 2, 1994). For example, a lens with transmission of 90 per cent in the faded state and 25 per cent in the darkened state would be described as a light/dark photochromic

Classification term	*Transmission (% at 25°C)*
Light	≥ 80
Medium	≥ 40 but < 80
Dark	≥ 15 but < 40
Extra dark	< 15

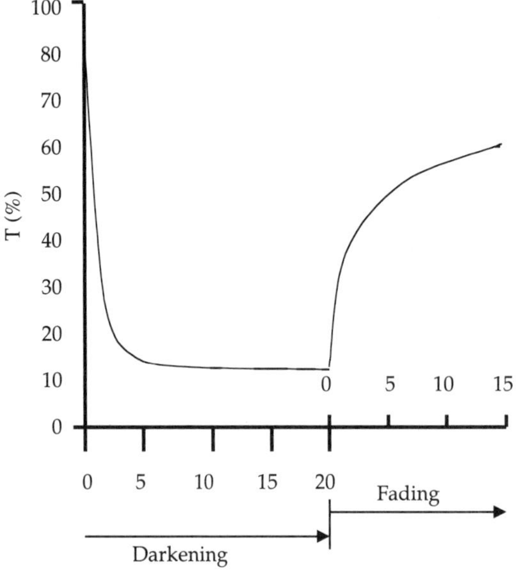

Figure 10.2. (a) Transmission performance of a glass photochromic lens. The graph shows a lens that initially transmits 100% of the incident light through it. On exposure to light the glass darkens, reaching a minimum transmittance of around 10% of the incident light after 5 minutes. When the lens is removed from the light after 20 minutes, it gradually fades towards its initial state. Note that even after 15 minutes fading the lens still only has a transmittance of 60%, as compared to its maximum original transmittance of 100%. (b) Transmission performance if a plastic photochromic lens.

example, a photochromic varying between 90 per cent and 25 per cent transmittance would be described as a light/dark photochromic.

Photochromics with a narrow variation in transmission between the faded and darkened states are promoted for use 'in the city', where light conditions change quickly between outdoors and indoors. These lenses maintain a pale tint in their faded state.

Photochromics with a wider variation in transmission between faded and darkened states are suitable for a narrower range of prescriptions, as the variation in the tint density across the lens is more apparent. These lenses also take longer to change between states than photochromics with a narrower variation in transmission, particularly with thicker lenses.

Photochromics are available in single vision, bifocal and varifocal forms. In fused bifocals, the segment is not tinted.

Laminated tints

Solid tints will vary in density depending on the lens prescription, so that a +6.00 D lens will transmit less than a plano in the same diameter, particularly in the thicker central part of the lens. This can cause problems in anisometropia, where the lenses will cosmetically appear to be different colours. Also, when prescribing tints the prescription must be considered along with the density of the material in order to obtain the required transmission. In order to overcome these problems, laminated tints (also described as equi-tints) are sometimes used, where a plano layer of solid tinted material is bonded to a powered component, which may be of high refractive index material if the prescription is significant. Such laminations naturally increase the cost of manufacture, and are sometimes thicker than a standard lens. One special purpose lamination, which has been used both for glass and plastic lenses, is where a polarizing tint is required. In this case, a sheet of plastic polarizing material is embedded between the front and back layers of a lens. Polarized lenses prevent plane-polarized light reflected from horizontal surfaces from entering the eye. As such, they are found useful by drivers, fishermen and skiers. Another special form of lamination uses a wedge-shaped cross-section of tinted material in order to give a darker tint at the top of the lens than at the bottom, known as a gradient tint.

Vacuum-coated tints

Solid glass tints have been largely replaced by thin film vacuum-coated tints. A thin metallic film is deposited by evaporation on to the rear surface of a spectacle lens in a vacuum chamber. This gives an even tint that is independent of prescription and lens thickness. A very wide range of colour options is possible, but the precise tint is difficult to reproduce at a later date, making single lens replacement problematical. The lenses should be considered purely as cosmetic unless transmission spectra are available.

Plastic lenses

Dipped tints

The standard method for producing tints on thermoset plastic materials (e.g. CR39) is to dip the lens into hot (80°C) dye – the dipped tint. In the simplest form of manufacture, the density of tint is controlled by visual matching against standard samples. This is an inexpensive and effective way of tinting, but is not easily reproducible unless more sophisticated control methods are used. Lenses should be supplied as matched pairs rather than individually, and should be regarded as being cosmetic in nature rather than providing specific protection unless transmission spectra are available. Gradient tints can be produced by slowly pulling the lens out of the tint bath, so that different parts of the lens are immersed for different periods of time.

Plastic photochromic tints

Plastic photochromic tints can either be solid, or moulded into the front surface of the lens only, as in the Transitions material (Figure 10.3). Chemically, plastic photochromics are totally different to glass, being based on organic dyes. Although many attempts were made to produce satisfactory lenses, it was not until the introduction of indolino spiroxazines in the early 1990s that lenses became available with a good fatigue life (Welch and Crano, 1992).

The speed of reaction is similar to that of glass materials (Figure 10.2), but it should be noted that plastic materials appear to require more UV radiation for activation. Plastic photochromics also show temperature dependency, going darker in cold temperatures.

Standards for tints

The minimum integrated visible transmission of a tint, or the mean transmission across the visible spectrum, is given the symbol τ_v. For general purpose use, the minimum value of τ_v that can be supplied in prescription form is specified in BS EN ISO 14889 (1997) as being 3 per cent. In other words, the maximum depth of tint is 97 per cent. Additionally, the spectral transmission at any wavelength in the range 500–650 nm should not be less than 0.2 τ_v. For driving, τ_v must be at least 8 per cent in daylight and 75 per cent at night. Specific requirements also apply to the visibility of traffic signals when lenses are used for driving. Separate requirements are

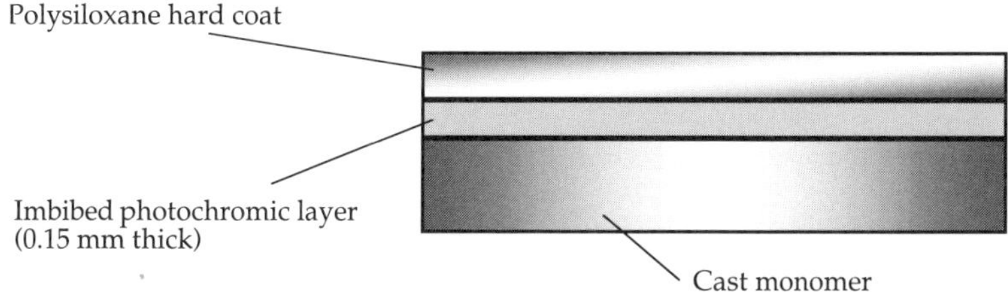

Diagram not to scale (from Norville/Transitions Optical)

Figure 10.3. The construction of a 'Transitions' surface photochromic plastic lens. The surface 0.15 mm of the plastic lens has been impregnated with the photochromic dye. A hard coating has been added on the surface of the lens.

laid down for non-prescription sunglasses, which are specified in BS EN 1836, 1997.

Treated lenses

Anti-reflection coatings

In order to reduce surface reflections from a lens and maximize transmittance of light through the lens, a thin film coating is applied in a vacuum chamber. The properties of this film must be very carefully controlled in order that it reduces reflections in the desired manner. These coatings were developed after it was discovered that glass telescope objectives that were some years old transmitted more light than identical ones that had been newly manufactured. The reason was found to be the atmospheric tarnishing of the surface layer of the glass changing the refractive index over a very thin layer.

The theory of anti-reflection coatings depends on light acting as a wave (Figure 10.4). If the reflected light from the lens has a wavelength λ, then if it is combined with light which is half a wavelength out of phase (λ/2 path difference), the two waves will destructively interfere,

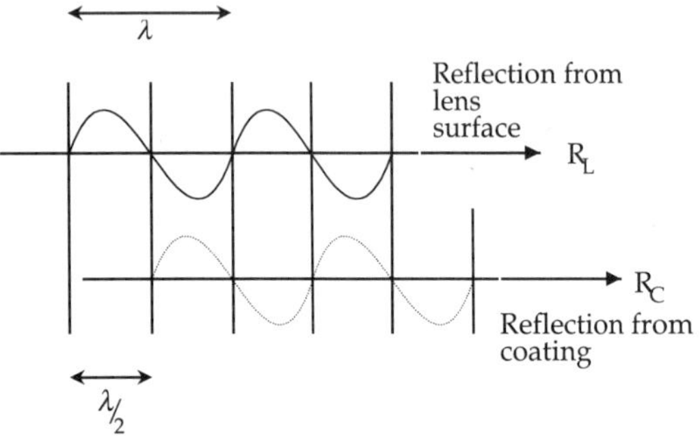

Figure 10.4. The use of destructive interference in the construction of anti-reflection coatings. The upper portion of the diagram shows a light wave of wavelength or spatial period λ, reflected from a lens surface. The lower portion of the diagram shows the reflection of the same light wave, of the same wavelength, reflected from a coating on the lens surface which is a distance of λ/2 from the lens surface. If the reflections from the lens and from the coating are summed, then it can be seen from the diagram that negative portions of one wave will be cancelled out by the positive portions of the other wave, and *vice versa*. The two waves are therefore said to destructively interfere, eliminating the reflection from the lens and coating surfaces.

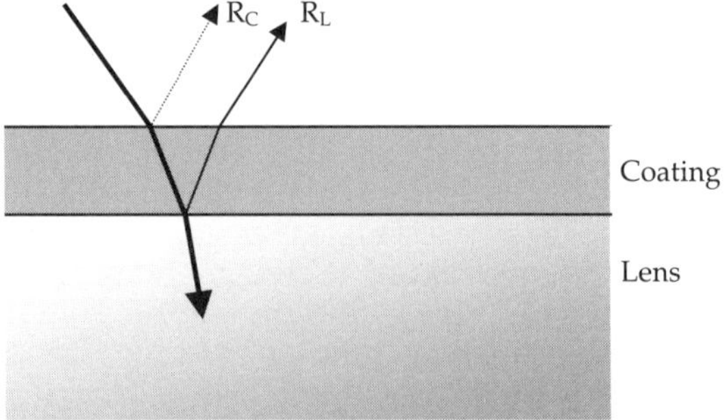

Figure 10.5. The diagram shows an anti-reflection coating on the surface of a lens. Light is reflected from both the coating surface (R_c) and the lens surface (R_L). In order to provide destructive interference, the distance the incident light ray must travel between entering the surface of the coating and leaving the coating having been reflected at the coating /lens surface junction should be λ/2. To achieve this, the thickness of the coating should be λ/4.

reducing the reflection to zero. Light not reflected is then transmitted. Thus in Figure 10.5, if a thin film is coated on the lens such that the extra path length of the light passing through the coating is half a wavelength, then interference will take place. As the light passes twice through the coating, the thickness should be half of $\lambda/2 = \lambda/4$. Hence the required thickness of an anti-reflection coating is one quarter of the wavelength of light.

The other optical property that needs to be considered in constructing an anti-reflection coating is the refractive index. For a lens of refractive index n' in a surrounding medium of index n, the reflection from a surface (σ) is given by:

$$\sigma = [(n' - n)/(n' + n)]^2 \qquad \textit{Equation 10.02}$$

Equation 10.2 gives a value for σ of between 0 and 1, where 0 indicates that no light is reflected at the surface and 1 indicates that all the incident light is reflected at the surface. The equation shows that reflectance increases with higher index lens materials. It also shows that reflectance is greater at the blue end of the spectrum, since any lens material has a higher refractive index for short wavelengths than for longer wavelength light (Chapter 1). If the amount of reflection from the coating/lens surface (σ_L) is made the same as the amount of reflection from the coating/air surface (σ_C), then the reflections will destructively interfere if the thickness condition discussed above is met. Thus for a lens material of refractive index n' with a coating of index n_c, in air, if:

$$\sigma_L = [(n' - n_c)/(n' + n_c)]^2$$

$$\sigma_C = [(n_c - 1)/(n_c + 1)]^2$$

and $\sigma_L = \sigma_C$

then

$$[(n' - n_c)/(n' + n_c)]^2 = [(n_c - 1)/(n_c + 1)]^2$$

taking square roots of both sides and expanding

$$(n' - n_c)(n_c + 1) = (n_c - 1)(n' + n_c)$$

$$n'n_c + n' - n_c^2 - n_c = n'n_c + n_c^2 - n' - n_c$$

$$2n_c^2 = 2n'$$

$$n_c = \sqrt{n'} \qquad \textit{Equation 10.03}$$

Thus the refractive index of the coating must be the square root of the refractive index of the lens material. For ophthalmic crown glass of index 1.523, this requires a coating of index 1.234. For a practical coating, there are two fundamental problems here. First of all, the theory shows that this coating is only effective at one wavelength of light, but spectacle lenses are used in conditions of broad band lighting across the full visible spectrum. Secondly, there is the problem of obtaining a coating material that is not only the correct wavelength, but is also durable enough to withstand the rough treatment given to spectacle lenses. Unfortunately, there is no material that satisfies these criteria fully. Magnesium fluoride ($n = 1.38$) is the most practical coating, despite having a less than ideal refractive index for many lens materials. However, for high refractive index materials, for example $n = 1.80$, it is much closer to the ideal value (which in this case would be 1.34).

More efficient coatings consist of several layers (Figure 10.6), which enables a lens to have reduced reflections over a wider range of wavelengths (Figure 10.7).

Practical benefits of an anti-reflection coating include that they:

- boost light transmission by reducing light lost at the lens surfaces by reflection
- reduce power rings (multiple internal reflections of the edge of a lens, particularly problematic to highly myopic spectacle wearers)
- reduce ghost images (faint images formed by reflection at the lens surfaces).

It is particularly important for high-index lens materials to be supplied with anti-reflection coatings, since a greater proportion of light is lost by reflection at the surfaces of these lenses compared to lower index materials.

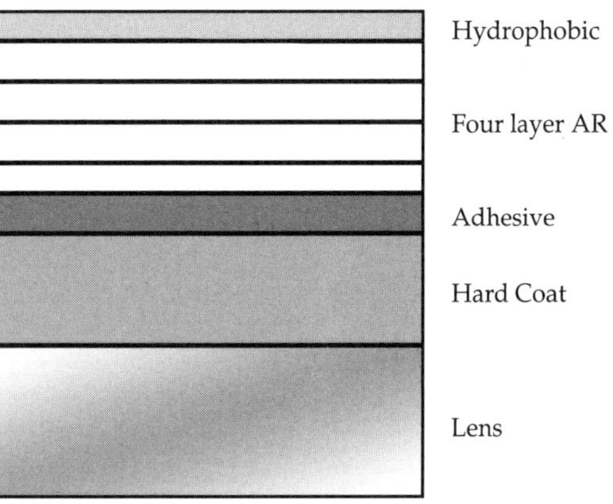

Figure 10.6. Cross-sectional view through a coated plastic lens (not to scale). The plastic lens substrate is coated with (in order): a hard, or scratch resistant, coat; an adhesive layer; four layers of anti-reflection coating to reduce reflections across a range of incident wavelengths; and a hydrophobic outer layer (after Wilkinson, 1996).

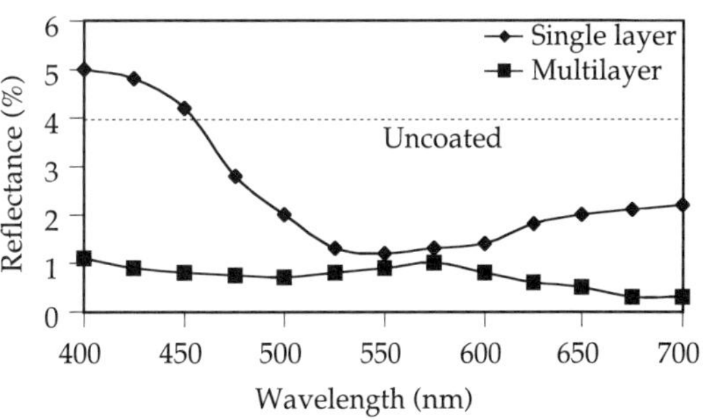

Figure 10.7. Reflection from one surface of a CR39 lens. In the uncoated state, reflectance at the surface is 4% (equation number 10.02). A single layer anti-reflection coating is effective at reducing reflections and improving transmission in one region of the spectrum (in this case, around 550 nm). A multilayer anti-reflection coating is much more effective at reducing reflections across the entire visible spectrum.

Scratch resistant coating for plastic lenses

Many plastic lenses are now supplied with a scratch resistant coating as standard. Although these coatings can be considered optional for thermosetting plastics such as CR39, they are essential for thermoplastic materials such as polycarbonate and acrylic. There is a problem with all hard coats, in that if they are too hard and inflexible they will crack under pressure or impact. In addition, it is difficult to get a coefficient of thermal expansion match between the coat and the lens substrate, which causes stress in the coating if the lens is subjected to extreme temperatures.

There are a number of different methods of application:

1. *Dipping*. Lenses are dipped into hard coat solution and the surplus material allowed to drain off. An example of the liquid hard coat is a mixture of alcohol pyrrolidone, acrylate ester and butyanol. As in all coating procedures, the lens must be scrupulously clean before coating takes place. This process is used in the mass production of lenses, but is not really suitable for coating straight top solid bifocals, as streaks of hard coat will form at the visible edge of the segment.
2. *Spin coating*. For small-scale production, a liquid hard coat is dripped on to the front of a lens on a spinning holder. The spinning action spreads out the coating evenly across the lens.
3. *Vacuum hard coat*. A silica coat can be deposited onto the lens surface in a vacuum chamber. This method requires expensive equipment, and the hard coat cannot be subsequently tinted. However, this type of hard coating is often used prior to the application of an anti-reflection coating.
4. *Hard coating 'in mould'*. This type of hard coat is introduced into the mould at the time of basic lens manufacture. The resultant lenses are difficult to tint, so the hard coat is usually only applied to the front surface of a lens. Hard coatings are typically 10–20 times thicker than an anti-reflection coating. Coating thickness and refractive index are critical, as unwanted interference effects, including enhanced surface reflections, may occur if the wrong combination is used.

Hydrophobic coatings

These are thin coatings applied to lenses to help keep the surfaces clean. The coating helps to prevent adhesion of liquid droplets, which will then fall off rather than dry out on the lens surface. They are particularly important for use with anti-reflection coatings, where any surface dirt is made more visible by the coating.

Safety lenses

When glass was the commonest spectacle lens material, it was recognized that the impact resistance of the material was not adequate for use in hazardous environments, or where accidental breakage was likely (for example by children). Thus various processes were developed to make glass lenses 'safer', which have broadly paralleled developments in glazing for cars and other vehicles. The use of safety lenses was given further impetus by the Food and Drug Administration in the USA, who introduced minimum levels of impact resistance, using a $^5/_8$ inch steel ball dropped from 50 inches, for all prescription lenses (except for a few special cases) in 1972. In Europe, BS EN ISO 14889 (1997) specifies a static loading test as a minimum safety requirement for any spectacle lens, where a lens must not break while a 100 N load is applied through a 22 mm steel ball for a minimum of 10 seconds.

Spectacle lenses for industrial use have separate impact resistance standards (BS EN 166, 1996).

Heat toughened glass

The process of manufacturing heat toughened glass involves heating up a finished, edged lens in an oven to 650°C, and then rapidly cooling the surfaces with cold air jets. The process was developed for spectacle lenses by Walter King of Cleveland, USA, in 1912. The heating time (50–200 seconds) is carefully controlled, and is related to the mass of glass and lens thickness. The resulting lens has a thin surface layer that is in a state of compression, and has a slightly different refractive index to the rest of the lens. The ensuing birefringence (difference in refractive error, dependent on the plane of polarization) gives rise to a characteristic 'Maltese-cross' pattern, which can be viewed through cross-polarizers (Figure 10.8). A non-toughened glass lens will show no pattern. Note, however, that localized stress patterns may be visible through a cross-polarizer, caused by tight glazing in metal frames, and that CR39 plastic lenses also exhibit considerable internal stress.

Lenses for heat toughening generally have to be made thicker than normal. Heat toughening has the advantage that it is quick and cheap, and is cost effective for small numbers of lenses. However it is not advised for lenses over ±10.00 D, rimless mounted lenses, fused bifocals and some types of solid bifocals. The process must be used with care on photochromic glass, as the heat cycle changes the colour of the tint as well as the response times.

(a)

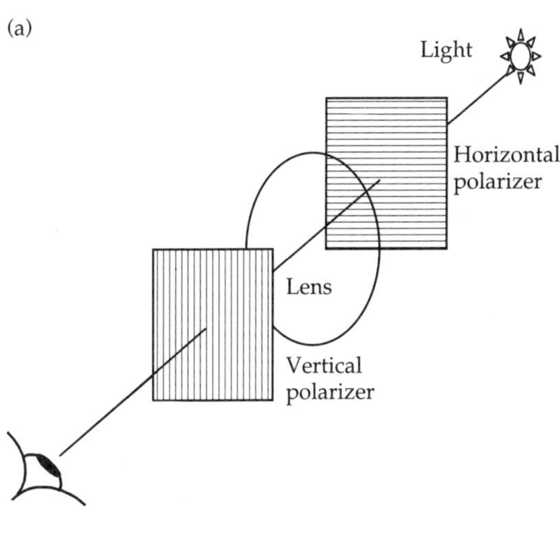

(b)

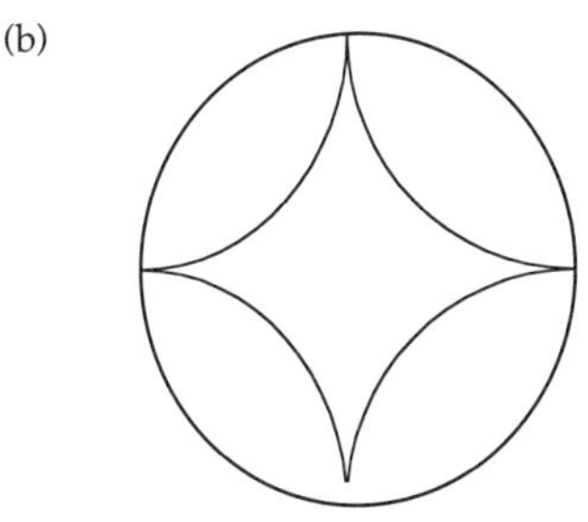

Figure 10.8. Identification of a heat toughened glass lens. When the lens is placed between two cross-polarizers (a), a characteristic 'Maltese-cross' pattern is visible on the lens (b).

Chemically toughened glass

The process for chemically toughening glass lenses was patented by Weber in 1965, and commercially developed by Corning Glass in 1971. The method consists of heating a lens for 16 hours in a bath of potassium nitrate at a temperature of 450°C. For photochromic glass, a mixture of 40 per cent sodium nitrate and 60 per cent potassium nitrate is used. The action of this process is to replace some of the surface sodium ions with potassium ions. Because the process takes place at lower temperature than heat toughening, there is less induced stress in the lens. Normal thickness glass lenses can be used. To verify chemical toughening, the lens must first be immersed in glycerine before viewing in a polarized strain tester, where a narrow band is seen around the periphery of the lens. A further technique has been developed to shorten the process by ultrasonic stimulation of the bath.

Chemical toughening has the advantage of using normal thickness lenses, but the long processing time and large number of lenses required to make a batch economic have meant that it has never been popular in the UK.

Laminated lenses

Unlike the toughening processes described above, laminated lenses do not have the aim of increasing the impact resistance significantly before the lens breaks. The object here is to retain the broken glass particles on a central plastic layer so that these do not enter the eye. To achieve this, two outer glass shells are bonded on to a central polyvinyl butyral plastic sheet.

Two attempts were made in the 1980s to update the lamination process. In one, a single layer of soft plastic was bonded on to the rear of a normal glass lens. In the other, the thickest component of the lens was the central plastic core, which had thin glass shells bonded to the front and rear, with the option of using photochromic glass.

All laminated lenses suffer from problems of edging into nylon supra and rimless mounts, and are prone to delamination in the long term.

Plastic lenses

All plastic lenses at 'normal' lens thicknesses are inherently more impact resistant than the equivalent untoughened glass lens. Figure 10.9 shows that the impact resistance of CR39 is better than that of toughened glass for the stated conditions. Note, however, that when CR39 does break it does so into very sharp slivers. CR39 and similar materials should not be supplied at normal thicknesses as 'safety lenses', but rather as 'break resistant lenses' in order to stress their limited impact resistance.

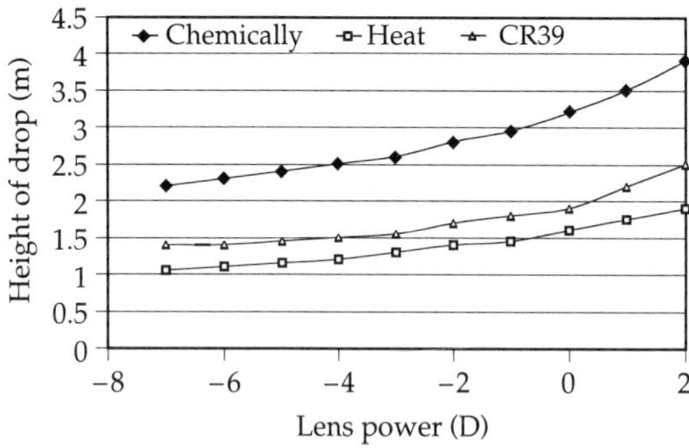

Figure 10.9. Impact resistance of lens materials across a range of lens powers. A 68-g steel ball is dropped onto the lens from various heights. The data points illustrate the maximum height from which the ball can be dropped and the lens remain intact. As expected from their greater centre thickness, more positive lenses are stronger than negative lenses. CR39 is seen to be stronger than heat toughened glass, and is certainly stronger than untreated glass. However, it is not stronger than chemically toughened glass. (After Corning, 1990)

Where significant impact resistance is required, the material of choice is polycarbonate. As shown in Table 10.3, this plastic is considerably more impact resistant than other materials, and is now available in a wide variety of prescription forms. As with other plastic lenses, environmental conditions may make glass a preferable choice – for example, in gritty environments or chemical laboratories. Polycarbonate is readily attacked by acetone.

Table 10.3 Impact resistance of various lens materials to a 6.5 mm steel ball (after Wigglesworth, 1972). The figures given for each material indicate how fast the steel ball must be moving to fracture a lens sample of the given thickness. It can be seen that polycarbonate has the most superior impact resistance

Material	*Thickness (mm)*	*Fracture Velocity (m/sec)*
CR39	2	39
CR39	3	49
Acrylic	3	34
Non-toughened glass	3	12
Heat toughened glass	2	12
Heat toughened glass	3	18
Laminated glass	3	12
Polycarbonate (coated)	3	152
Polycarbonate (uncoated)	3	244

Summary

In this chapter, the coatings available to incorporate with spectacle lenses have been discussed. Tints to reduce the transmission of light through a lens can be supplied in various ways, either by incorporating the tint with the lens material, which can lead to difficulties in variation of tint with lens thickness, or by surface treatment. Tints can be supplied in fixed or photochromic form. Other coatings that can be added to spectacle lenses include anti-reflection and scratch resistant coatings. Finally, the various forms of safety lens have been discussed.

Formulae

Formula	*Name*	*Equation number*
Density = $1/(\log T)$	Tint density	10.01
$\sigma = [(n' - n)/(n' + n)]^2$	Reflectance at a lens surface	10.02
$n_c = \sqrt{n'}$	Refractive index of AR coating	10.03

Appendix: Useful websites

1) British Standards Institution
(www.bsi-global.com)
Provides an online list of all current British standards, and is particularly useful for finding the latest version of a standard.

2) Delphion Intellectual Property Network
(www.delphion.com)
Comprehensive search facility for US, European and Japanese patents. Particularly useful for up-to-date developments in progressive lenses and lens materials.

3) Butterworth-Heinemann/*Optician*
(www.optometryonline.net)
Site giving news and developments in optometry, dispensing and manufacture, as well as information on books and publications in the ophthalmic field.

References

Adams, A. J., Kapash, R. J. and Barkan, E. (1971). Visual performance and optical properties of Fresnel membrane prisms. *Am. J. Optom.* **48**, 289–97.

Alvarez, L. W. and Humphrey, W. E. (1970). Variable power lens and system. US Patent No. 3 507 565, US Patent Office, Washington DC.

Aves, O. (1907). Improvements in and relating to multifocal lenses and the like, and method for grinding the same. UK Patent No. 15 735, Patent Office, London.

Baker, T. Y. (1943). Ray tracing through non-spherical surfaces. *Proc. Physical Soc.* **LV**, 361–4.

Bennett, A. G. (1965). The true founder of point focal lens theory: George Biddell Airy. *Optician* **50**, 422–5.

Bennett, A. G. (1970–71). Variable and progressive power lenses. *Optician* **160**, 421–7, 533–8; **161**, 10–22.

Bettiol, B., Harsigny, C. and Lenne, W. (1981). Ophthalmic lens series having an aspheric surface. US Patent No. 4 279 480, US Patent Office, Washington DC.

BS 2738–1 (1998). Spectacle lenses – part 1. Specification for tolerances on optical properties of mounted spectacle lenses. BSI.

BS 2738–3 (1991). Spectacle lenses – part 3. Specification for the presentation of prescriptions and prescription orders for ophthalmic lenses. BSI.

BS 3062 (1985). Specification for ophthalmic lens materials. BSI.

BS 3521–1 (1991). Terms relating to ophthalmic optics and spectacle frames – part 1. Glossary of terms relating to ophthalmic lenses. BSI.

BS 3521–2 (1991). Terms relating to ophthalmic optics and spectacle frames – part 2. Glossary of terms relating to spectacle frames. BSI.

BS 7394–2 (1994). Complete spectacles. Specification for prescription spectacles. BSI.

BS EN 166 (1996). Personal eye-protection. Specifications. BSI.

BS EN 1836 (1997). Sunglasses and sunglare filters for general use. BSI.

BS EN ISO 7944 (1998). Optics and optical instruments – reference wavelengths. BSI.

BS EN ISO 8429 (1997). Graduated dial scale. BSI.

BS EN ISO 8598 (1998). Optics and optical instruments – focimeters. BSI.

BS EN ISO 8624 (1997). Measuring system for spectacle frames. BSI.

BS EN ISO 9342 (1998). Optics and optical instruments – test lenses for calibration of focimeters. BSI.

BS EN ISO 14889 (1997). Fundamental requirements for uncut spectacle lenses. BSI.

Charman, W. N. (1991). *Visual Optics and Instrumentation*. Macmillan Press.

Corning (1990). *The Handbook of Ophthalmic Glass*, UK edn. Corning France Optical Division.

Davis, J. K. (1979). The dotting lens. *J. Am. Optom. Assoc.* **50**, 591–4.

Davis, J. K. and Fernald, H. C. (1965). Ophthalmic aspheric lens series. US Patent No. 3 169 247, US Patent Office, Washington DC.

Evans, B. J. W. (1997). *Pickwell's Binocular Vision Anomalies: Investigation and Treatment*. Butterworth-Heinemann.

Fowler, C. W. (1984). Aspheric spectacle lens designs for aphakia. *Am. J. Opt. Physiol. Opt.* **61**, 737–40.

Fowler, C. W. and Sullivan, C. M. (1990). Automatic measurement of varifocal spectacle lenses. *Ophthal. Physiol. Optics* **10**, 86–9.

Freeman, M. H. (1990). *Optics*. Butterworth-Heinemann.

Jalie, M. (1980). Ophthalmic spectacle lens. UK Patent Application No. 2 030 722, UK Patent Office, London.

Katz, M. (1982). Aspherical surfaces used to minimize oblique astigmatic error, power error and distortion of some high positive and negative ophthalmic lenses. *Appl. Optics* **21**, 2982–91.

Okada, T., Nakamura, T., Nakamura, K. *et al.* (1986). Spectacle lens. UK Patent No. 2 163 864A, UK Patent Office, London.

Smith, G. and Atchison, D. A. (1983). Construction, specification, and mathematical description of aspheric surfaces. *Am. J. Opt. Physiol. Opt.* **60**, 216–23.

Sullivan, C. M. and Fowler, C. W. (1988). Progressive addition and variable focus lenses: a review. *Ophthal. Physiol. Optics* **8**, 402–14.

Tunnacliffe, A. H. and Williams, A. T. (1985). The effect of vertical differential prism on the binocular contrast sensitivity function. *Ophthal. Physiol. Optics* **5**, 417–24.

Tunnacliffe, A. H. and Williams, A. T. (1986). The effect of horizontal differential prism on the binocular contrast sensitivity function. *Ophthal. Physiol. Optics* **6**, 207–12.

Volk, D. and Weinberg, J. W. (1962). The Omnifocal lens for presbyopia. *Arch. Ophthal. NY* **68**, 776–84.

Von Rohr, M. (1909). Spectacle glass. UK Patent No. 15 533, UK Patent Office, London.

Welsh, R. C. (1978). Spectacle lens for aphakia patients. US Patent No. 4 073 578, US Patent Office, Washington DC.

Whitney, D. B. (1958). An automatic focusing device for ophthalmic lenses. *Am. J. Optom.* **35**, 182–90.

Welch, C. N. and Crano, J. C. (1992). Plastic photochromic eyewear: a revolution. In: *Ophthalmic Visual Optics Technical Digest*, vol. 3, pp. 13–16. Optical Society of America.

Wigglesworth (1972). A comparative assessment of eye protective devices and proposed system of acceptance testing and grading. *Am. J. Optom.* **49**, 287–304.

Wilkinson, P. (1996). Ophthalmic lenses and dispensing. *Optician*, **212** Part 10, July 19, 24–32; **212** Part 11, August 16, 32–37.

Woo, G. C., Campbell, F. W. and Ing, B. (1986). Effect of Fresnel prism dispersion on contrast sensitivity function. *Ophthal. Physiol. Optics* **6**, 415–18.

Index